Improving The Odds

From The Crapshoot Of Manipulative Therapy

To

The Innate Chiropractic Adjustment

Robert Clyde Affolter, D.C.

Improving The Odds

From The Crapshoot Of Manipulative Therapy
To
The Innate Chiropractic Adjustment

Published by Robert Clyde Affolter

For information, please contact:
Innate Foundation
www.innatefoundation.com

Printed in the United States of America
February 2002 Edition

Dedication

Each person on this planet has been sent here with a mission. When the physical and mental interference to Innate expression has been removed, the person accomplishes the mission flawlessly. Some people have been sent here with the mission of removing the interference to Innate expression. They measure their success not in dollars or numbers of patients seen, but in the satisfaction received each time the imprisoned Innate impulse has been completely released. We call those people CHIROPRACTORS and it is to you this book is dedicated.

Table of Contents

Preface

This book is an ongoing work. It is designed to provide a taste of the logic and reason of chiropractic, plus a taste of our scientific heritage. It is not intended to be a scientific or scholarly work – it started out that way but a friend's advice was that it was too short, terse and uninteresting. The real change came because it wasn't fun for me. The result is this book of my experience. It is written pretty much like I talk. The grammar may not always be perfect – but I think you will find it more interesting.

We are all entitled to our opinions and by writing mine down you are welcome to have them. My opinions are based on 47 years of experience as a patient (my father was a chiropractor) and 17 years of practice.

When I was a kid we got checked every once in awhile no matter how we felt. If we didn't feel good, we got checked more often. I don't remember any pattern to it (once a week, once a month, or what). I remember getting checked one day, thinking I felt fine, and needing an adjustment. Immediately after the adjustment, I felt my forehead relax as though I had been frowning and not aware of it. I found that pretty interesting. You could feel fine and get an adjustment and feel even better!

Until I was about 15 my father practiced out of our house. When I was around 9, I remember a little girl used to come around the house to play with us after she was checked. She was quite cross-eyed. By the time we were in junior high school, you could hardly tell she was cross-eyed at all. That is one example of my experience.

At one point I developed low back pain. I was about 11 years old. Dad said my problem was in my neck, but adjusting my neck wasn't helping. After a couple of weeks he finally x-rayed my neck to see what was going on. I can still remember him smiling as he held the x-rays up to the light and said, "I've been adjusting the wrong side." I was well the next day. That experience convinced me that your neck could cause low back pain and that x-rays were important.

My father died in 1979. My mother and I spent one morning giving patients their records. One man stayed to tell me his story. He had fallen off of a scaffold and had become quite debilitated. When the local doctors couldn't do anything they sent him to the University of Kansas School of Medicine. After over a week of testing, they sent him home and told him he would get the results in the mail. They told him he had a rare disease and would never work again. However, when they sent him home he went to see Dad and was already working when he got their diagnosis.

The point is that I had some idea of what health problems chiropractic was good for (all of them) before I went to chiropractic college. While attending Palmer College of Chiropractic, I became interested in the upper cervical approach (partially because I knew it had been the foundation of my father's work). I found the upper cervical chiropractors to be some of the best thinkers in our profession. I still believe that upper cervical chiropractic is the best way to start your chiropractic career.

I believe upper cervical chiropractic epitomizes the philosophy, science and art of chiropractic. While this book goes beyond upper cervical adjusting, I continue to use the scientific, philosophic approach I developed as an upper cervical practitioner.

By the way, I know some think that upper cervical chiropractors are under educated followers of a dogma that should have been buried long ago. My resume is included in the back of the book (for those impressed by degrees acquired by sitting on your butt in classes). For those who are not impressed by degrees but are impressed by the force of a logical argument, I offer to debate anyone, anywhere, anytime (as long as it fits my schedule and you pay my fee - which I keep reasonable – I debate mainly for the entertainment).

Please keep in mind as you read this book that I agree that any technique that corrects a subluxation gets sick people well. I also agree that no matter what you do and how good the technique, everyone will die eventually. I only encourage you to be the best you can be.

*"The only failure a man should fear,
is the failure to do his best."*
D. D. Palmer

Introduction

I remember Dr. Crowder giving a guest lecture to the Upper Cervical Society when I was a student. After all these years, I don't remember the exact words so I will give my version of part of his lesson and change it to speak to you right now. Imagine that we are meeting in a room, on the second floor of the library building at Palmer College of Chiropractic.

Each of you is in one of two conditions – you are either subluxated or you are clear. If we would go to the top of the stairs and push you down the stairs, when you land at the bottom you would be in one of three states – improved, worse or no change. What we are trying to do is improve on those percentages.

How about you? What percentage are you satisfied with?

My father was a chiropractor. I was always impressed with his simple logic. He believed that an adjustment had to be specific. A friend of his once said that he didn't believe in specific adjustments – he just loosened everything up and let Innate put them back. Dad's reply was an offer to hit the doctor in the mouth and let Innate straighten his teeth.

I grew up with the idea that x-rays were important. X-rays told how to adjust and skin temperature analysis along with leg checks told whether to adjust or not. Chiropractic was simple. Dad said, "Quacks do something different to everyone. I do the same thing to everyone and they all get well."

Too many in our profession have gotten over educated with the result that fewer people are getting well. A common comment I have heard is that a person is a wonderful doctor – his adjustments didn't help but he referred me for massage, gave me vitamin supplements, etcetera, etcetera. The goal of this book is to give a powerful yet simplified method of practicing chiropractic – that gets results.

Some believe that if the patient's symptoms change then correction must have been accomplished. However, they often also believe that if symptoms don't change it's not the fault of the chiropractor – the patient just needs nutritional supplements, massage, exercise, drugs or surgery.

There is a growing faction among our ranks who realize that if we are to get superior results we must correct the subluxation. As chiropractors look more to proving that the subluxation has been corrected (using technology such as thermography and EMG), the importance of accurate adjustment of the upper cervical area will become obvious.

Years ago I offered to take x-rays for chiropractors in my area. I had a precision aligned double L frame, head clamps and locking chair. One of the other chiropractors sent a kid for neck x-rays and after developing them I checked them for quality. The misalignment was so obvious that I remember thinking "this is an easy one." A few weeks later I got the x-rays back in the mail. The x-ray envelope had the return address of one of the orthopedists in town. The kid hadn't gotten better and had been sent for orthopedic consultation.

We all have difficult cases. One of my instructors said that a subluxation misalignment might be as small as the thickness of a sheet of paper. This book will not make you an upper cervical specialist, capable of finding minute misalignments; that is not my goal. It is my goal to help you find the big misalignments and to come up with a rational approach to delivering an adjustment; thereby increasing your results and decreasing orthopedic referrals.

The book is divided into parts. Part One will cover chiropractic philosophy. I will present my views on explaining Innate Intelligence as Life, speculate on the electromagnetic nature of the universe and the human condition, and give my idea of the game of life.

Part Two will focus on the science of chiropractic. In Part Two, I will cover the importance of the upper cervical subluxation, the physics of the upper cervical misalignment, x-ray analysis and the physics of the adjustment.

The art of chiropractic will be covered in Part Three. I will present a patient encounter from initial consultation to post adjustment examination and some ideas on report writing and practice management.

In Part Four, I will review some of the chiropractic techniques that have had the most effect on my practice. The reviews are designed to be brief introductions and sources are listed for more information.

> *"Chiropractors do not 'heal,' they are not 'healers': salves heal. They do not 'cure,' charms cure. Medicines cure by virtue of the hidden magic contained therein."*
>
> *D. D. Palmer*

Part 1: Philosophy

Chiropractic is a **philosophy**, science and art. The philosophy explains why we do what we do as chiropractors. Without a solid understanding of philosophy, chiropractic is reduced to the mere manipulation of joints. In this part of the book, I will look at chiropractic philosophy and give my opinions and ideas on our unique profession.

"The New Theology enunciated by me more than ten years ago as the basis of Chiropractic, is the identification of God with Life-Force. The Intelligent Life-Force of Creation is God. It is individualized in each of us. It desires to express itself in the best manner possible.

In every phase of life, vitality and action, man's highest aspiration should be to advance himself to a higher level, to make himself better mentally and physically.

God - The Universal Intelligence - The Life-Force of Creation - has been struggling for countless ages to improve upon itself - to express itself intellectually and physically higher in the scale of evolution."

D. D. Palmer

Is There Really An Innate Intelligence?

Several years ago, I helped organize a car pool for local chiropractors to go to our state capitol. On the ride home, I talked with a young chiropractor who said he did not know if there really is such a thing as Innate Intelligence. I was appalled. Here was a practicing chiropractor who had no idea, no understanding, and therefore no confidence in the profession of which he professed to be a part.

I have no intention of trying to recreate a complete chiropractic philosophy text here. However, let's look at the question: Is there an Innate Intelligence?

Archeologists dig up artifacts and make inferences about ancient civilizations. For example, they might find a bowl made of clay and they conclude that the culture knew how to make a bowl out of clay and they might even speculate as to how the culture used the bowl. I hear no arguments that the bowl just evolved, on its own, from clay.

If we look at the evolution of the automobile, from the old horseless carriage to the present day computerized, climate controlled vehicles we see the enormous advancement in engineering. I hear no arguments that the automobile just evolved, on its own, from iron ore.

The reason we don't hear those arguments is that we don't believe that matter, such as iron ore or clay, is capable of forming something without the intelligent guidance of man. Yet, when we look at life processes, which are even more complex than automobiles, some say life just evolved without intelligence. I ask you to be consistent. If something as complex as a human body can evolve without an intelligent guiding force, then so can an automobile, a bowl or any other invention.

What is intelligence? I define intelligence as an ability to adapt to new situations. Can life adapt? Certainly. Does your body build antibodies to organisms that it has never seen before? Usually. Does your body digest food it has never tasted before? Usually. Does your body eliminate poisons by vomiting, diarrhea, etcetera? Usually.

Notice that all the answers are usually. It is more likely that your body will adapt than fail to adapt. Now, which is more intelligent your Innate Intelligence, which you were born with, or your Educated Intelligence, which you have gained from experience and schooling?

One day a patient came in and complained of nausea and diarrhea. I checked her and scheduled another appointment. She said that she thought she should see her medical doctor. I said go ahead. Next time she came in I asked her if she went to the M.D. She said, yes. The conversation went something like this:

"What did he say?"

"He said I have an intestinal virus."

"What did he propose to do about it?"

She rummaged in her purse and produced two bottles of pills. Holding a bottle of pills in each hand, she said, "He gave me this bottle for nausea and this bottle for diarrhea."

"Yeah, that's why I could never be a medical doctor."

"What do you mean?"

"Well, let's assume that he's right. You have an intestinal virus. Your body is trying to eliminate the virus by throwing it out both ends and he's going to keep it in there. It just makes no sense."

Educated Intelligence often wants to control the symptoms and disregards Innate without even thinking. It is up to the chiropractor to look to Innate and make sense of the condition.

People have looked for the cause of diseases for centuries. Chiropractors look for the cause of health. Innate Intelligence is the cause of everything in the body.

Want some examples?

Many people think exposure to the sun is the cause of sunburn. Yet a corpse will not sunburn. The effects we call sunburn are the response of Innate Intelligence to the sun. Do you need to read studies published in medical journals to tell you that getting a sunburn is a bad idea? Or can you take the pain that your own Innate gives you as the signal?

What about smoking? Does smoking cause cancer and other diseases? Based on the research I have seen, I remain unconvinced. Is smoking a good idea? Hand a boy a cigarette and have him inhale. Isn't the cough Innate's rejection of the smoke? Wouldn't that tell us that it is probably not a good idea to smoke? That people can adapt and eventually smoke without coughing is further evidence of Innate's ability to adapt.

We are taught that diseases are caused by bacteria and viruses. Inject a corpse with a virus or bacteria and you will find none of the signs and symptoms of disease. Again, the signs and symptoms are the result of Innate Intelligence.

Some may agree but find that this discussion is not useful. The problem is we have not been taught to apply our philosophy. Look at AIDS. A person can be HIV positive and not have AIDS. Why not? Innate is adapting to the organism without creating the condition known as AIDS. Our question is: Does the body stop adapting successfully because of a subluxation?

There is an Innate Intelligence running your body right now. If you can, take a moment and stand up, then stand on one foot, and sit down. As a chiropractor, you might be able to write down all of the tendon attachments, nerve supply and blood supply for all the muscles used to perform those tasks. However, do you realize that it would take a physicist quite a while to figure the exact pull on each of those muscles to keep you balanced? Can you appreciate that a young child, with no knowledge of physics or anatomy, can perform the tasks just as well as you?

It makes sense that there is an Innate Intelligence running every cell of your body. It coordinates your body to function in harmony or ease. Innate controls the body, primarily, by using the nervous system. Cells send messages to the brain using nerves. Innate then uses nerves to send messages back to the cells to keep the body in harmony.

Interference to those messages going to the brain or coming from the brain result in a lack of harmony or dis-ease. The vertebral subluxation (a bone in the spine which is misaligned and impinging the nervous system) creates interference and results in dis-ease.

An adjustment corrects the subluxation, removes the interference, restores transmission of messages from Innate and given time ease is restored.

It is important for the chiropractor to fully understand the above steps. Much of the research coming out today is not based on the philosophy of chiropractic and is therefore bunk!

For example, a surgeon and I got into a letter writing debate. He complained that chiropractors do no research and nothing we did had ever been proven effective. He then did some research and found a study purporting to show that chiropractic was no more effective than a placebo for a certain kind of headache. He sent me a copy while gloating that chiropractors had done research and proven that our procedures were no more effective than placebo.

The procedure was to provide spinal manipulation of the neck twice per week for four weeks and assess the outcomes. The placebo control was massage of the neck. Nowhere in the report was there any mention of adjustments holding and a patient not being manipulated. After explaining the chiropractic philosophy to the surgeon, I pointed out that we had no idea whether the manipulations were actually adjustments (meaning nerve interference had been removed). We had no idea whether any of the manipulations actually subluxated the patients. We further had no idea whether the massage reduced subluxations or created them. Therefore, based on the chiropractic premise and philosophy the study was worthless.

I then asked him what placebo was used to convince him that appendectomies were a valuable treatment.

The surgeon never responded to that letter.

How about you? Do you know your patient is subluxated before you thrust? What are your criteria? After you thrust, do you know if your thrust was a manipulation or an adjustment? What are your criteria?

The better your criteria for finding a subluxation – the better you will find subluxations. The better your adjustments – the better you will clear your criteria. The better you clear your criteria – the fewer adjustments you will perform. The fewer adjustments you perform – the better your patients will become.

If you have been telling patients the importance of weekly adjustments, I encourage you to change your vocabulary. Weekly adjustments cannot be justified philosophically, scientifically, or even emotionally. The idea of weekly adjustments is utter nonsense. Now, weekly checkups, an examination to determine whether a patient is subluxated or clear, make sense. Ideally we will refine the science and art of chiropractic to the point where every person will get only one adjustment, unless they have a new trauma. In addition, ideally, every person will understand the importance of periodic chiropractic checkups to ensure that they do not need an adjustment. Although both of those ideals seem unlikely, they certainly give us something to work toward.

"To express the individualized intelligence which runs all the functions of our bodies during our wakeful and sleeping hours, I chose the name Innate. Innate - born with."

D. D. Palmer

Chiropractic vs. Medicine

As I read an article written by B. J. Palmer, the developer of chiropractic, I thought of our current situation. The article was written in 1959 and is just as appropriate today. The public is sick and desires to be well. They have two choices – medicine and chiropractic. The choices differ greatly. Which should they pick? The choices can't both be right or can they?

Dr. Palmer stated that the medical profession is right in their approach to the treatment of diagnosed diseases and the chiropractic profession is right in their approach to correcting the cause of dis-ease. How can both be right? It is like a two-lane highway.

If you were to take a two-lane highway from New York to Los Angeles you would be safest on the right side of the road. If you took the same highway from Los Angeles to New York, you would again be safest on the right side of the road. In both cases you would be right because your destination was in opposite directions. The choice is similar between chiropractic and medicine – you must know your destination.

The medical profession has no concept of health other than feeling good and not dead. Therefore, any treatment that prevents death or makes you feel better is considered appropriate.

The chiropractic concept of health is based on the concept of an Innate Intelligence. If you cut yourself, you were born with an ability to heal yourself. You were born with an ability to make antibodies when you get an infection. The very definition of intelligence is the ability to deal with new or trying situations. The fact that you were born with that ability means that the intelligence is innate. The chiropractic concept of health starts with this statement: The one cause of health is Innate Intelligence.

Some choose to debate that one statement. What about nutrition, exercise, rest, a clean environment? If you have no Innate Intelligence (life), you cannot digest your food, move muscles, sleep or enjoy your environment. Without Innate Intelligence you are dead and your body decomposes to the soil from which it came.

If you have an Innate Intelligence, why are you sick? Your Innate Intelligence uses your brain and nervous system to control your body. If a bone in your spine puts pressure against a nerve (directly or indirectly), it interferes with the electrical signals from your Innate Intelligence. Your body is then not properly controlled and becomes out of balance. Dis-ease is the condition of your body when it is out of balance. If you are in a state of dis-ease, you are sick.

An adjustment replaces the vertebra, restores the nervous system, removes interference to the electrical signal, and puts your Innate Intelligence back in control, which restores balance and restores health. Can any medication do that?

As always, the choice is up to you. Do you want your disease treated or your health restored? If you choose to have your disease treated, you must realize that ultimately the medical doctor is counting on that same intelligence to make you better. Eventually the doctor throws up his hands and says, "We have done all we can do. It is up to Nature now." They call Innate Intelligence – Nature.

The chiropractor realizes that it was up to Nature, Innate Intelligence, all along. If you choose to have your health restored, will you keep it restored with periodic checkups to make sure the nervous system is free of interference? Those checkups are health care.

Can we have the best of both worlds? Can we use chiropractic care and medical care? When they are not in conflict it would make sense. It makes sense to have chiropractic care after surgery so that the incision heals properly. It makes sense to have chiropractic care after a bone is set so that it heals properly. It makes sense to have regular chiropractic checkups no matter what your condition or how you feel.

"Students of Chiropractic should constantly remember that disease is not a thing, but a condition. It is abnormal performance of certain morphological alterations of the body."
D. D. Palmer

Chiropractors – What Makes Us Different?

What is the cause of disease? Nobody knows. But many think they have an answer. Confusion runs rampant. Which disease? What is the diagnosis? There is no such thing as disease. The founder of our profession, D. D. Palmer, stated, "… disease is not a thing, but a condition." Disease is a loss of appropriate function. If appropriate function returns we say the disease was cured and health has returned.

Now if I change the question to: What is the cause of appropriate function? Confusion still exists but not quite so rampant. Suddenly everyone goes, "Huh?"

For most of the population, health means I am not dead and I feel okay. The dictionary often defines health as optimum function and lack of disease. I prefer to say health is the ability to adapt to changing conditions. Health is appropriate function. Let's forget about the confusion of terms between health and disease. What is the cause of appropriate function – Innate Intelligence! That is what makes us unique. It is the only platform on which we must stand.

My daughter came in for dinner one night after playing with her friends. After a few minutes she began vomiting. I asked her what she had eaten. She said that she and her friends had made stew. She had taken carrots and the other kids had picked beans off of the trees. The "beans" were poison pods. To the average person my daughter was sick. However, a quick call to poison control told us that vomiting was the appropriate response. If she was not vomiting we were to give her ipecac! She wasn't sick – she was healthy! Her body was functioning normally and adapting to the environment.

Let's look at my daughter's condition and try to think our way through the process. She ate something poisonous. It apparently did not taste bad or if it did she swallowed it anyway. Something somewhere decided that what was in her stomach was harmful to her body and needed to be expelled. That decision appears to be a sign of intelligence. After all, my daughter's body (at the age of five) had reached the same decision as the doctors at poison control. The nervous system receives signals from the stomach as to the contents of the stomach and Innate makes decisions based on the information received. Innate determined that a poison was in the stomach and sent messages, via nerves to the stomach, causing contractions of the muscles to expel the poison.

Let's look at another similar example. When I was about seven, I attended a family picnic and drank too much soda pop. After a three-hour car ride, I felt awful, but I did not vomit. My father checked me and determined that I needed an adjustment. He adjusted my atlas and called to my mother to bring a bucket. My mother barely made it into the room before I started vomiting. What happened? I had an atlas subluxation. The nervous system's messages from my stomach to my brain or from my brain to my stomach were not working properly. I felt sick and from a chiropractic standpoint I was not in a state of health, because I was subluxated. Once the subluxation was corrected, the mental impulses were restored, normal function returned; the body recognized the poison and eliminated it. I vomited – appropriate function – health restored. Chiropractic is as simple as that and that is what makes chiropractors different.

Retracing - What Is Innate Doing?

The body is under intelligent control. When it seems to be out of control, it is our job to figure out what Innate is doing. A subluxation interferes with the nervous system and Innate's messages to control the body. However, we must remember that Innate will strive to make the best of the situation by adaptation and compensation.

Treatment of a patient's symptoms makes the patient feel better and may be quite important in some cases; but it has long been the chiropractic argument that treatment of symptoms without correcting the cause is not health care. By that, we mean that the subluxation must be located and corrected to correct the cause of the condition. Failure to correct the subluxation leaves the patient sick, no matter what change in symptoms has occurred.

With the above in mind, let's look at what happens to our subluxated patient. For the sake of argument, let's assume we start with an atlas subluxation. A common complaint might be headache, but there may be no symptom at all. Due to the interference at the brain stem, the muscles to the lower back are affected. We check the patient and find a short leg due to the muscle imbalance. Left uncorrected, the body begins to adapt and compensate for the subluxation. Innate changes the curve in the neck in an attempt to reduce the interference at the brain stem.

As the body adapts, the symptoms change. Over time, the headaches may disappear and lower back pain may develop. Innate continues to adapt. The lower back develops a curvature in an attempt to relieve the nerve interference at that level. Now the thoracic area is under stress and indigestion is the complaint.

When the subluxation is adjusted the adaptations are no longer needed and Innate must go through the process of correction. It often happens in reverse order. In our example, first the thoracic area would straighten and indigestion would improve. The lower back may then hurt. The low back curvature straightens and headaches return. Finally, all adaptations are removed and the headaches are gone.

The reversal of symptoms during the healing process is known as retracing. Retracing is a specific chiropractic explanation for a common clinical pattern. It is not an excuse for hurting patients and making them worse.

My first experience with retracing was as a chiropractic student. I had an elderly patient who had been experiencing back pain for over thirty years. After several weeks of care, her back seemed a little better, but she noticed a return of migraines which she had not had since she was a teenager. The migraines were not as severe as in her youth and only lasted a few days, but were a classic example of retracing.

By the way, when I was graduating I introduced this patient to her next student doctor. As we reviewed her complaints, she stated that her allergies were also better, I teased her that she just finally "outgrew" them (after over 70 years.) The new student doctor said that maybe the pollen count was lower this year. She said that her friends' allergies were just as bad as ever and she thought her improvement was due to her chiropractic care. This person had been quite skeptical when she started and I did not tell her that her allergies would get better. She drew those conclusions on her own.

That is how we have traditionally "sold" chiropractic, with RESULTS.

Research

Chiropractors often blame lack of federal money and ostracism by the medical community for the lack of chiropractic research. The situation is improving. Medical researchers and chiropractors are working together.

However, most chiropractors are unaware of the research which has been done. B. J. Palmer established a research clinic and hired a medical staff to determine the effects of chiropractic care on various medical diagnoses. Although the research was done prior to the knowledge of statistical analysis, his protocol was fascinating.

Patients were examined by both medical and chiropractic facilities. Neither was allowed to talk to the other. Palmer wanted to determine if sick people could get well simply by finding and correcting vertebral subluxations. He did not want the chiropractor's decisions altered by the medical diagnosis. He took the research a step further, by not allowing the medical doctors to see their original diagnosis. Palmer published the research findings; showing changes in vision, hearing, blood values, and urinalysis.

Although not valid by today's statistical standards, I point out that it has been estimated that as little as 15% of modern medicine has been proven using statistical analysis. When I couple that estimate with the knowledge that even when medicine is proven statistically effective, it is often of questionable practical value, I am quite comfortable with our scientific footing.

For example, if 5% of a given population is at risk, and medication could reduce their risk to 1%, is that justification for medicating 100% of the population? From a chiropractic philosophical perspective, it is not. Medicine is interfering in the lives of 95% of the population, and making them sick, because medical doctors can't determine whether a given individual is in the 5% at risk group or the 95% group not at risk.

This kind of research is weak and unsuitable to the clear, precise thinking of chiropractic. We must be on guard when we work with our medical brethren that we not fall into their treatment mentality. Chiropractic research is a different beast.

The chiropractic questions are: Is the person subluxated? If the person is subluxated, what effect is the subluxation having on the person's health? If the subluxation is corrected, what effect does the adjustment have on the person's health?

Once again I reiterate, in any chiropractic research project, the first phase must be to establish criteria for determining that a subluxation exists. The prospective subjects must then be examined for subluxation. Those who are clear can be used as a control. Those who are subluxated, but not adjusted, can also be used as a control. Those who are adjusted are the experimental group. Everyone, in every group, must be examined regularly using the subluxation criteria to determine if subluxation exists.

By the end of the study, some in the clear control group may be found to be subluxated and must be excluded. Some in the subluxated control group may be found to be clear and must be excluded. Some in the experimental "adjusted" group may be found to be subluxated, meaning the subluxation was never corrected, and must be excluded. Without regular examination of all participants, the research will be worthless, based on our philosophy.

We would predict that people in the clear control group who later became subluxated would do poorly. We would predict that people in the subluxated control group who became clear would do better. We would also predict that people in the experimental "adjusted" group would do poorly, if their subluxations were not actually adjusted/corrected.

The ideas that the harmful effects of a subluxation stem from nervous impingement and that the beneficial effects of an adjustment stem from removal of nervous impingement are what separate the science of chiropractic adjusting from physical therapy's manipulation. Careful and rigorous adherence to those ideas will not only help our profession progress, but will help delineate worthless therapies from valuable chiropractic service.

"The ultimate objective of EVERY adjustment MUST be to increase size, shape, diameter and circumference of all occlusions, to release all pressures, to correct all interferences and to restore all transmissions whether that be between occiput and atlas, atlas and axis or to replace odontoid process of axis into normal situ, to give freedom to passage of spinal cord without pressure, to permit a normal free full 100% quantity flow of mental impulse supply between brain and body; to release brain congestion above and release body starvation below."
B. J. Palmer

Vaccination

Many chiropractors are opposed to vaccinations. They question the actual effectiveness of the vaccines and point to the people who have been harmed by the procedures. Other chiropractors agree with the medical profession or believe that the issue isn't worth fighting.

It is not the position of chiropractic to be anti-medicine. It is a duty of every person to question public policy and encourage those things which have a positive benefit and discourage those things which are harmful.

From a philosophical perspective, vaccination introduces toxins into healthy people while failing to make sick people healthy. A sick person is sick because he is subluxated. Even if the vaccination were 100% effective and harmless, there is very little reason to believe that the vaccination will correct the subluxations of those who are sick. So, while leading people to believe that they are protected from disease and therefore healthy, they are actually only protected from one organism and still sick.

For example, let's say 10% of a population would die from the flu because of a weakness of their immune system due to their subluxations. If the vaccine was 100% effective, and we knew which 10% would die, we would vaccinate them and they would not die from the virus for which they were vaccinated. However, their immune systems are still weak and susceptible to other viruses and bacteria. The sick people were not made healthy.

Unfortunately, the vaccines are never 100% effective, nor harmless. Nor do we ever know which 10% are actually going to die from the flu. So, everyone is vaccinated. Everyone is harmed, to some extent. Perhaps worst of all, the sick are never found and made healthy.

It is this slipshod method of applying "health care" to the community, which runs against our philosophy. The community is not sick. Individuals are sick. The community does not need treatment. Individuals need adjustment.

We should raise questions regarding the effectiveness of vaccinations. We should question the harm vaccinations may be doing. More importantly, we should be checking people for subluxations and adjusting sick people back to health. As each individual becomes healthy, the health of the community improves.

"Vaccination and inoculation are pathological;
Chiropractic is physiological."
D. D. Palmer

Accumulative Constructive or Destructive Survival Value

We are constantly changing and adapting. Are the changes positive and constructive or negative and destructive? The medical profession is constantly looking for something outside the body which correlates with early death. Cigarette smoking has been said to have a destructive effect on the body. We also believe that the damaging effects of cigarette smoking are cumulative. In other words, the more cigarettes a person smokes, the more destructive the effect.

Similar effects seem to be true of alcohol consumption, usage of drugs, poor diet, and various types of physical abuse of the body. The effects are cumulative.

What about a subluxation? What are the effects? If a subluxation exists, interference to the normal adaptive processes of Innate exists. The body is out of harmony and the effects are negative and cumulative. Given time, the lack of harmony will accumulate to the level of a recognizable alteration of physiology. It will be said that disease exists. The patient may be symptomatic or asymptomatic.

If the subluxation is adjusted, Innate's normal adaptive process is restored. The effects are positive and cumulative. Given time, the body will return to harmony and it will be said that the disease was "cured."

In between are most cases. The subluxation is adjusted but recurs. Part of the time Innate is in control and the process is positive. Part of the time Innate is being blocked and the process is negative. If the negative process lasts longer than the positive process, the case is getting worse. If the positive process lasts longer than the negative process, the case is getting better.

Until 1930, it was generally believed that a subluxation had to be adjusted daily for weeks or months to make a correction. B. J. Palmer's research proved such not to be the case. According to Palmer, a subluxation was not a subluxation 24 hours per day – even if not adjusted. Therefore the cumulative effect was not as predictable as might be thought.

Dr. Palmer claimed that the on again – off again nature of a subluxation explained the up and down nature of disease processes; for example, the rise and fall of fever during the course of a day. It also explains the seeming efficacy of some medications. Aspirin taken for a headache, when a subluxation exists, may depress the nervous system and relieve pain until the subluxation is not a subluxation and the headache has disappeared.

What makes a subluxation a subluxation? Certainly the misalignment must interfere with the nervous system. However, what if the interference is below the level of Innate's ability to adapt? If Innate adapted to the reduced capacity of the nerve, it would be possible that the patient could still be healthy. Let me give you two analogies, one using a car and the other a computer.

My wife took our car to a mechanic for a tune-up. When I got home she said that she smelled gas while she was driving. I planned to take the car to a seminar the next day, so I got a flashlight and looked at the engine. The mechanic had replaced the gas line filter going into the carburetor. The line was leaking at the connection, so I tightened it. I drove the car around the block and smelled no gas. All seemed fine.

The next morning I left early for the seminar. The car ran fine all the way through town, but when I accelerated to get on the freeway it nearly stalled. I drove for over an hour and a half. The car ran fine unless I tried to pass someone. Then it would almost stall.

I looked at the engine but could see nothing wrong and took it back to the mechanic and explained the problem.

He found that when I tightened the gas line I twisted it. The kink was under a covered part of the line, so I couldn't see it. The kink would not let the normal amount of gasoline to the engine. As long as I was going a constant speed, there was enough fuel in the reserve bowl of the carburetor. As soon as I hit the accelerator, the carburetor would go dry because the feed was not fast enough.

A similar situation happens with computers. A high speed modem will work well on a good phone line. However, if the phone line is degraded, the modem will slow down to get the data through correctly. As long as speed is not needed the situation might go unnoticed. If the speed of the connection is critical, the interference cannot be tolerated.

Could it be that the body is the same? Is it possible that the person with indigestion, who does fine on a bland diet, is compensating for nerve interference? Is it possible that once the nervous system is corrected the stomach could handle nearly any food and would respond as quickly as my car once the gas line was fixed? How many people are babying themselves and cannot live their full potential because of a subluxation?

The understanding of when a subluxation exists (meaning nerve interference is present) and needs an adjustment is one of the hallmarks of post 1930's chiropractic. The daily "adjusting" of the spine with no idea of whether nerve interference exists at the moment of adjustment is an old chiropractic idea, which is ready for the trash heap.

"...whether the case is growing better or worse depends upon HOW MUCH OF THE TIME THE VERTEBRAL SUBLUXATION IS PRESENT OR ABSENT, whether it be a minority or majority of the time, and whether bad works faster per hour than good can repair or balance per same time involved."

B. J. Palmer

Electromagnetic Communication – Innate's Radio

Let's look at the operation of a radio in simple terms. The radio station, a transmitter, sends an electromagnetic vibration. The radio uses energy, usually provided by a battery or wall outlet, to create a vibration. When the vibration of the radio matches the vibration of the radio station, the speaker vibrates and produces sound.

Is the human body very different from a radio? The eye detects electromagnetic vibration in the form of light and sends the vibration to the brain. The ear detects electromagnetic vibration in the form of sound and sends the vibration to the brain. Pressure and temperature sensors also are recording vibrations and sending the vibrations to the brain.

Is it possible that our bodies are sophisticated radios? Is it possible that we use the food we eat for energy to cause the proper vibration? Is it possible that the nervous system is the wiring or circuitry of our radio? Is it possible that each person has a unique frequency that Innate Intelligence uses to control the body by sending and receiving vibrations?

The answers to those questions seem to be yes. Chiropractors fix the short circuits in the nervous system wiring. What about tuning the vibration?

Many in our profession think we should expand the practice of chiropractic. They would include diagnosis, medications, exercise, etc. What should be the basis of our expansion?

I am including this chapter to provoke thought. If the simple radio analogy is true, chiropractic is certainly the basis for all healing. A radio will never function properly if the circuits are not right. What about tuning? Does the body automatically adjust its frequency once the nervous system is clear? Could the proper frequency allow the transmission of mental impulses to muscles and correct the vertebral subluxation?

Our philosophy should direct our research. The questions in this chapter could provide the basis for chiropractic research that would build on the work of B. J. Palmer and put chiropractic solidly at the forefront of healing science. How does Innate communicate with the body? What interferes with Innate communication?

Those questions inspire me. Whether chiropractic is an effective treatment for back pain or headaches does not. How about you?

"Nerves have no channels; their carrying capacity depends upon their ability to vibrate. Normal vibrations carry the normal amount in a natural manner."

D. D. Palmer

The Game of Life

What do you do for amusement? Play a game? Watch a movie? One day I watched my son playing a computer game. He was intensely being the character on the screen. The computer game experience is similar to watching a movie. He sits and watches the screen. However, the game is interactive and seems to change based on what he does. Once he beats the game he is tired of it and ready to play something else. The experience started me thinking about life and the things we do to amuse ourselves.

Many people are writing or talking about a Oneness in the universe. Is there a Universal Intelligence of which we are all a part? If so, why were we created?

Imagine, if you can, that you are the Universal Intelligence. You are all that exists. There is nothing to do. You are bored. You decide to amuse yourself. Why not create a game? So you begin to create a game similar to the computer game my son was playing.

First, you create a universe in which to play the game. Then you create creatures to play the game. The creatures have senses such as sight, smell, hearing, touch, and taste and you create a world that stimulates the senses with a full range of experience from beautiful landscapes with fragrant flowers, to desolate desert with scorching sunlight.

Then you give the creatures emotions such as joy, sorrow, love and hate. You make each creature unique with strengths and weaknesses, special talents and abilities. Each creature has certain experiences it desires for joy and love and other experiences that give pain and sorrow. You give each creature its own Innate Intelligence, a unique part of your Universal mind, which keeps the creature in existence as it plays the game.

Now you are ready to play and as you become each creature you forget that you created the game. You forget who the characters are. You actually forget how to play. For each creature is given another intelligence – its Educated Intelligence. The Educated Intelligence starts from zero at birth and learns to play the game. The Educated Intelligence eventually believes that *it* is all-powerful, that *it* is in control, that the universe responds to *its* desires.

Yet for all its power, its ability to manipulate the environment with machines, its ability to manipulate its body with drugs, its ability to clone animals and alter genetics – it still must ultimately realize that it has no power. Without life (Innate Intelligence) the body has no reaction to drugs. Without life animals cannot be cloned and altered genes have no effect. No matter how carefully the Educated Intelligence manipulates the world, Universal Intelligence can wipe out the Educated creation with a minor hurricane, tornado or volcanic eruption.

Indeed the Educated Intelligence must ultimately learn that it has no power, it is simply part of an elaborate, exquisite game – a game it cannot win for it has no power. As we surrender we find that in losing we win! For as we surrender, we once again know the Creator of the game. We once again remember who we are and become Innate Intelligence – that unique expression of Universal Intelligence. Those who have given up the Educated and become Innate are known as Innate men or women.

Innate men and women play the game a little differently. They respect Innate knowledge over Educated guesswork and seek to perfectly play the part which they created - to enjoy the full range of sensations and emotions – and yet stay balanced and centered.

Next time you play a game or watch a movie think about YOUR life, YOUR movie, YOUR game and appreciate all the ups and downs – the comedies and tragedies – for there really is no better amusement.

"Some few men possess the INNER 'AWARENESS' to let THE INNER GREATER intellectuality come thru to the lesser, darker outer fellow and shed its 'light'…
…WITHIN EVERY LIVING PERSON is this same Innate personality that is the GREAT I AM THAT I AM."

B. J. Palmer

Part 2: Science

Chiropractic is a philosophy, **science** and art. The science of chiropractic explains how we do what we do. In this part we will look at the anatomy and physics of the upper cervical subluxation and how to correct it.

"Some Chiropractors waste much time using adjuncts. If this time was utilized in studying the principles of Chiropractic and their application, the profession would be advanced. Adjunct users should read and study Chiropractic literature; but, these are the ones who do not care to advance…. Chiropractic is a science just so far as it is specific."

D. D. Palmer

The Upper Cervical Area – Why So Important?

The key to understanding the importance of the upper cervical area is the recognition of the effect a subluxation of atlas or axis can have on the medulla oblongata/brain stem/spinal cord. Once the neurology is understood, the broad sweeping claims made by upper cervical practitioners become not merely plausible but simple common sense.

Anatomists state that the brain stem stops at the foramen magnum and becomes the spinal cord. Yet, the anatomic structure of the nervous tissue does not change instantly as it leaves the skull. Consult any good anatomy text and you will see that the medulla oblongata/brain stem/spinal cord could be directly affected by the narrowing or distortion of the spinal canal caused by misalignment of atlas relative to occiput and axis. Also note the extension of the nuclei of the cranial nerves and the possibility of affecting those nerves. Then look at the arrangement of the spinal cord itself. Notice that the motor tracts going to the lower limbs are on the outside of the cord and most easily affected by distortion of the spinal canal.

Indeed, a leg check is usually cleared with an upper cervical adjustment. Why? The muscles in the lower back are pulling the pelvis asymmetrically due to nerve interference at the cord. Once the subluxation is corrected, the nerve interference is removed, the muscles pull symmetrically and the pelvis is balanced. Think about it. If the pelvis is misaligned, as evidenced by the leg check, and an upper cervical adjustment corrects the misalignment, as evidenced by the leg check, hasn't the entire spine been affected?

A chiropractor once asked me what I tell people when they come in with low back pain and I am going to adjust their neck. I replied that I examine them and tell them my findings. Then most people will go along with a gag and let me adjust them. Then they feel better and figure I know what I'm talking about. He said, "Just results, huh?" I always wondered what he was telling patients if it wasn't based on results.

Next consider the autonomic nervous system and the organs controlled by it. The general chiropractor often looks at specific vertebral levels with influence being sympathetic or parasympathetic and the organs that might be affected by the specific level. Indeed, charts have been created depicting the various organs and nerve supply.

However, the upper cervical specialist recognizes that the brain gives specific influence over the autonomic system via the spinal cord. Therefore, rather than look for whether a condition is sympathetic or parasympathetic and whether the subluxation is a third dorsal or sacrum, the upper cervical chiropractor looks at the upper cervical area as the possible cause of interference to both sympathetic and parasympathetic systems.

Once you have reviewed the anatomy and physiology of the brain stem and spinal cord, you may still wonder if upper cervical misalignment can affect the cord. Dr. John Grostic proposed the Dentate Ligament Cord Distortion Hypotheses. In essence, he stated that the dentate ligament is attached to the pia mater and the dura mater. The dura is attached to the foramen magnum, atlas and axis. Misalignment of the atlas relative to occiput and axis would pull on the dura, and in turn pull on the dentate ligaments and distort the cord. We will also look at the distortion of the bony ring of the spinal canal in the next section.

I have found that when chiropractors focus too much on relating anatomy and physiology to the patient's presenting condition they wind up performing a medical diagnostic workup rather than a chiropractic analysis. The questions are always: Is the patient subluxated? If the patient is subluxated, where is the misalignment? How can correction be facilitated (the adjustment)? Lastly, has the subluxation been reduced or corrected?

"The difference between knowing WHERE, WHEN, AND HOW, and not knowing, makes the difference between success and failure."
B. J. Palmer

The Upper Cervical Misalignment

It is helpful if you get an articulated occiput, atlas and axis set. Understanding the shape and relationship of the bones is key to understanding the misalignments, palpating misalignments, seeing the misalignments on film, and correcting the subluxation with an adjustment.

Take your occiput, atlas, axis set and move the bones so that the joints are aligned with maximum clearance for the cord. Hold the occiput so that the posterior portion is closest to you and look down through the skull. Notice that the condyles converge anteriorly. Notice the position of the dens. Position the dens in the fovea dentalis of atlas. The space between the dens and the atlas lateral masses (interodontoid gap) should be the same on both sides. Notice the relative positions of the posterior rings of atlas and axis. (Illustration 1)

Now rotate the bones and look at them as though you were looking at a lateral film. (Illustration 2) Have the anterior of the bones facing to your left. Hold the atlas and axis in your left hand with a finger on the anterior tubercle of atlas. Place gentle pressure on the occiput with your right hand (simulating the weight of the skull) and move the occiput anteriorly on the atlas. You should see the atlas teeter with the posterior arch rising toward the occiput. (Illustration 3)

You have just created a posterior misalignment of atlas. Relative to the condyles the atlas has moved posterior. Some would call this an anterior occiput. This has also been described as an inferior atlas, indicating that the anterior tubercle of atlas is inferior to its normal position relative to the posterior arch. I will continue with the Palmer listing and call this an inferior atlas (AI – inferior.) What we call it is unimportant as long as we understand the physics of the misalignment. The atlas is posterior compared to its neutral relationship to the condyles.

Now move the occiput posterior, while still holding the pressure simulating the weight of the skull. The posterior arch of atlas should teeter toward axis. (Illustration 4) You just created an anterior misalignment of atlas, which could be called a posterior occiput, or a superior atlas. I will call it a superior atlas (AS – superior.) The atlas is anterior compared to its neutral relationship with the condyles and the anterior tubercle is superior compared to its normal position relative to the posterior arch.

Look at the bones from posterior to anterior. Note the convex shape of the condyles that fit into the concavity of the atlas. The condyles converge to the anterior and the convergence will be seen on the APOM (anterior to posterior open mouth) x-ray as a change in density. See the distinctive concavity in the occiput between the condyles and follow the concavity from the midline to the medial inferior portion of each condyle. Center the atlas under the occiput making sure that the joint surfaces match. (Illustration 5) Notice the internal aspect of the lateral masses should be equal distance from the center point between the condyles.

While holding pressure down on the occiput, slowly move the occiput to the left. You should note resistance to the lateral movement caused by the left condyle bumping against the left lateral mass of atlas. A steeper, deeper, or more concave lateral mass will create more resistance than a flatter, shallower or less concave lateral mass.

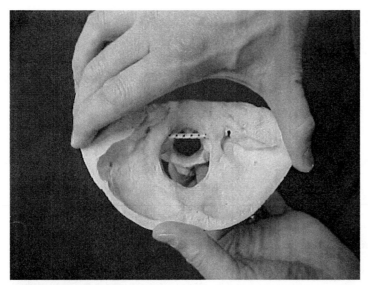

Illustration 1
Occiput, atlas and axis viewed from superior.

Notice the alignment of the bones to allow maximum room for the brain stem.

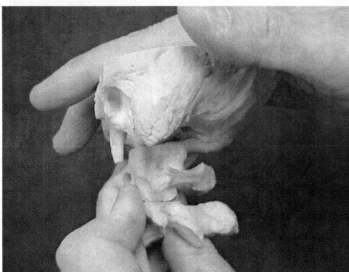

Illustration 2

Lateral view
Occiput, atlas and axis

The atlas posterior arch splits the distance between the occiput and the axis.

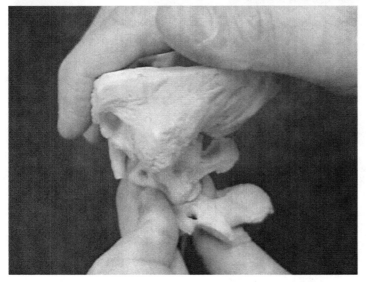

Illustration 3

Lateral view
Occiput, atlas and axis

AI atlas – the atlas has moved posterior relative to the condyles, the posterior arch of atlas is closer to occiput than the spinous of C2.

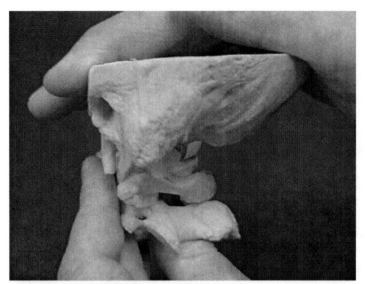

Illustration 4

Lateral view
Occiput, atlas and axis

AS atlas – the atlas has moved anterior relative to the condyles, posterior arch of atlas is closer to the spinous of axis than the occiput

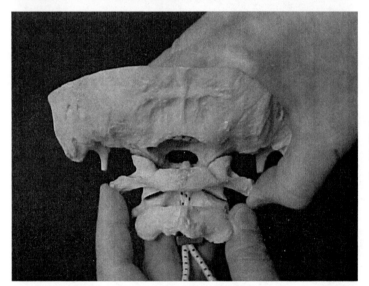

Illustration 5

Posterior view
Occiput, atlas and axis

Align occiput, atlas and axis to allow maximum room for the brain stem. Note the relationship of the structures.

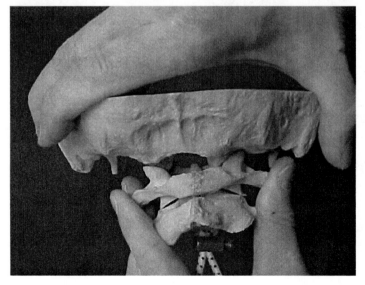

Illustration 6

Posterior view
Occiput, atlas and axis

Right atlas sideslip - AR

Note the right transverse process is closer to the occiput than the left transverse process. Compare the medial aspects of the lateral masses to the condyles.

Allow the occiput to pivot into the atlas so that the right side of the occiput slides inferior into the atlas and the left side of the occiput slides superior out of the atlas. (Illustration 6) You have just created a right lateral sideslip of atlas, or a left lateral sideslip of occiput. I will call this a right atlas (AR – right.) Notice that the right atlas has the left medial aspect of the lateral mass closer to the midpoint between the condyles. The right atlas also has the right transverse closer to the skull. If you were to draw lines across the inferior tips of the condyles and the inferior tips of the lateral masses, you would see the lines converge on the side of atlas laterality (providing there is no malformation of the condyles or lateral masses.)

Try moving the right condyle anterior and left along the right lateral mass. Relative to the condyle the atlas has moved right and posterior and will show up as an AI atlas on the lateral film. (Illustration 7) Now, try moving the left condyle posterior and left along the left lateral mass. The atlas is moving right and anterior relative to the condyle and will show up as an AS atlas on the lateral film. (Illustration 8) We have just created three right misalignments of atlas: right on both condyles, tracking posterior on the right condyle - AIR and tracking anterior on the left condyle - ASR.

Move the occiput to the right and create a left atlas sideslip - AL. (Illustration 9) Move the left condyle anterior and right along the left lateral mass and create the left posterior atlas - AIL. (Illustration 10) Move the right condyle posterior and right along the right lateral mass and create the left anterior atlas - ASL. (Illustration 11)

Now hold the occiput and rotate the atlas in the transverse plane. As you rotate you will again notice resistance caused by the concavity of the lateral masses and that both condyles ride up superiorly on the lateral masses. A deeper concavity will offer more resistance to rotation. Rotation can best be evaluated on a base posterior or vertex film. For our purposes, we will ignore rotation.

We can now describe eight misalignments of atlas, all will begin with A (atlas anterior to axis): AR (right), AL (left), AS (superior), AI (inferior), ASR (superior and right), ASL (superior and left), AIR (inferior and right), AIL (inferior and left.)

Let's look at axis. Axis cannot move anterior relative to atlas due to the dens hitting the anterior arch of atlas. (Illustration 1) For the same reason, atlas cannot move posterior relative to axis. Any misalignment of atlas relative to axis will be anterior. Which is the reason all atlas listings begin with A and all axis listings begin with P in Palmer's listing system. Relative to the atlas and the spinal canal the axis body can move laterally right or left and the spinous can move right or left.

Once again hold the bones so that you are looking at them from the posterior. Hold the axis body midline and move the spinous to the left. (Illustration 12) You must rotate the axis to perform that movement. Notice the C2/C3 joints. As axis spinous moves left, the left inferior articulating surface must move anterior and superior relative to C3, or C3 would misalign with axis. You now have an example of axis PLS (posterior to atlas, spinous left of body and superior on the left.)

Create an axis PRS (posterior to atlas, spinous right of body and superior on the right) by holding the body centered and moving the spinous right. Notice the interodontoid space (the dens is still centered) and notice the distortion of the spinal canal caused by the posterior ring. (Illustration 13)

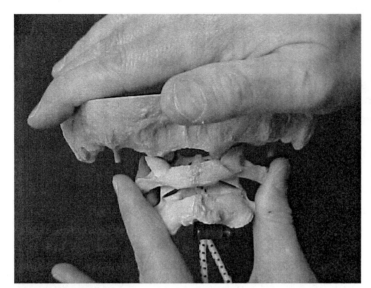

Illustration 7

Posterior view
Occiput, atlas and axis

Right posterior atlas - AIR

As the atlas moves posterior on the right condyle the posterior arch approaches the occiput.

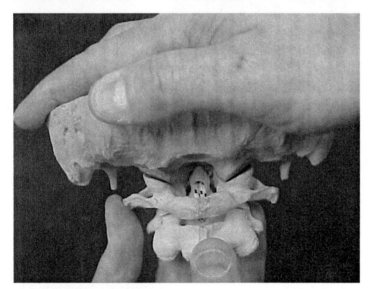

Illustration 8

Posterior view
Occiput, atlas and axis

Right anterior atlas - ASR

As the atlas moves anterior the posterior arch moves away from the occiput and toward the spinous of axis.

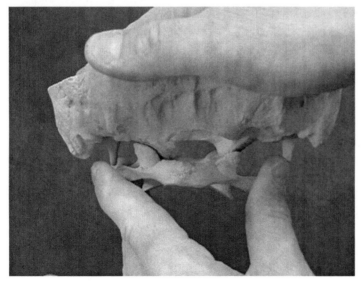

Illustration 9

Posterior view
Occiput and atlas

Left atlas side slip - AL

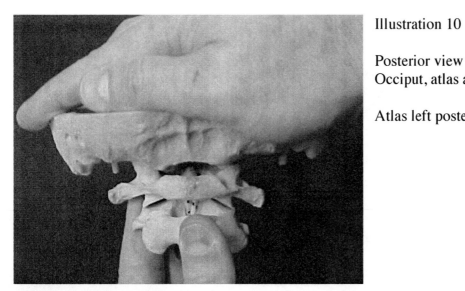

Illustration 10

Posterior view
Occiput, atlas and axis

Atlas left posterior - AIL

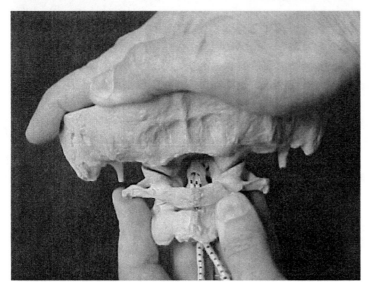

Illustration 11

Posterior view
Occiput, atlas and axis

Left anterior atlas - ASL

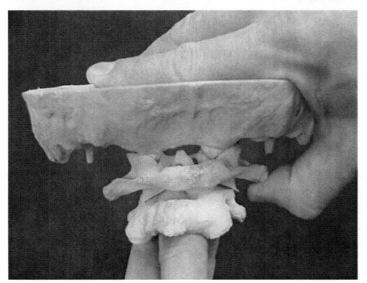

Illustration 12

Posterior view
Occiput, atlas and axis

Axis spinous left - PLS

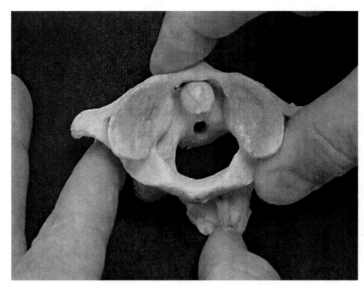

Illustration 13

Superior view

Atlas and axis

Axis spinous right – PRS

Interodontoid space – space between dens and the lateral masses are equal on both sides.

Try holding the spinous midline and moving the body of axis to the left. (Illustration 14) Notice again the joints between C2 and C3. The body of C2 must move posterior and inferior on the left relative to C3 (or C3 would misalign with axis.) You now have a body left axis. Move the axis body to the right to create a body right. As you move the axis, once again notice the interodontoid space. The dens is not centered. (Illustration 15)

Now keep the axis spinous in the center of the body and move the entire vertebra to the right. The interodontoid space is now smaller on the right (like a body right) and the spinous is also right of the midpoint between the condyles, but the spinous is centered relative to the axis body. This is an entire segment right axis. (Illustration 16) Create an entire segment left by moving the axis to the left while holding the spinous centered relative to the axis body. (Illustration 17) For this to happen with no rotation, occiput and altas must move together.

Rarely, axis may stay centered and move straight posterior – P. We now have seven listings for axis: P, PL, PR, body left, body right, entire segment left, and entire segment right.

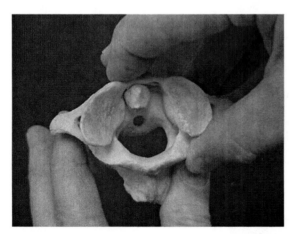

Illustration 14

Superior view

Atlas and axis

Axis Body Left - BL

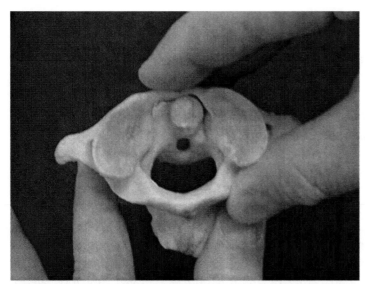

Illustration 15

Superior view
Atlas and axis

Axis Body Right - BR

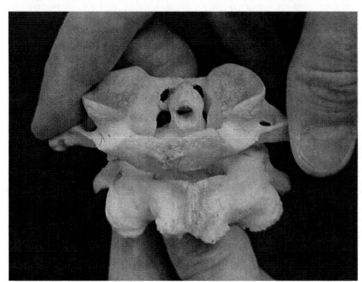

Illustration 16

Posterior view
Atlas and axis

Axis entire segment right

ESR

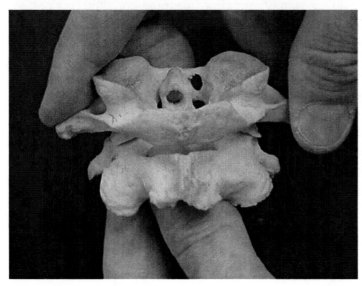

Illustration 17

Posterior view
Atlas and axis

Axis entire segment left

ESL

X-ray Analysis

Now that we have covered the misalignments with the bones, we will see what they look like on film. First look at the lateral. Draw or visualize the plane lines across the foramen magnum, atlas and axis. (Illustration 18, 19, 20) Do we have an AI atlas? Does the atlas plane line converge posteriorly with the foramen magnum line? Is the posterior arch of atlas closer to the occiput than the spinous of C2? (Illustration 21)

Or do we have an AS atlas? Does the atlas plane line converge with the foramen magnum line anteriorly? Is the posterior arch of atlas closer to the spinous of C2 than the occiput? (Illustration 22)

Next look at axis. Is the dens pointed posterior into the spinal canal? (Illustration 23) Are the C2/C3 joints aligned or can you see both left and right sides? As axis rotates you will often see both the right and left joints on the lateral, but if it is straight the joints will overlap and appear as one joint, or it will be difficult to see two sides. (Illustration 22)

When analyzing the Anterior to Posterior Open Mouth – APOM, first look at the condyles. Find the medial portion of the condyles and the center point between them. It may be helpful to use a ruler to find the center of the condyles.

Look for an atlas sideslip. If necessary, go back to the misalignment section and review.

Is the atlas centered under the condyles? Look at the medial portion of the lateral masses. Is one lateral mass closer to the midpoint between the condyles than the other lateral mass? Compare the medial aspect of the condyles with the respective lateral mass. Do they appear matched or is one side more medial and the other side more lateral (the right lateral mass would be more lateral if it is right of its condyle and the left lateral mass would be more medial if it were right of its condyle.) Can you tell if the condyles converge or are more parallel? Does one side of the atlas appear to be superior (approaching the skull) compared to the opposite side? (Illustration 24, 25, 26)

Next, compare the midpoint of the condyles to the axis. (Illustration 26) Is the dens centered under the occiput (in other words under the midpoint?) Is the spinous centered? If the spinous is right or left of the dens, is the body of axis elevated on the side of the spinous (PLS or PRS?) (Illustration 27) If the dens is right or left of the midpoint between the condyles, is the body of axis low on the side of laterality (meaning body left or right?)

Last compare the atlas to the axis. If the atlas is centered to the occiput (APOM) and the axis is centered to the atlas, the listing is determined by the lateral (AS or AI atlas or P axis.)

If the atlas is centered and the axis is misaligned relative to the condyles, is your finding consistent with the relationship of atlas to axis? In other words, if the dens is left of the condyles and atlas is centered, then the interodontoid gap on the left should be smaller than the right. If the atlas is centered and the dens is right of the condyles, then the interodontoid gap will be smaller on the right.

If the atlas is right of the condyles, is it also right of the axis? Compare the interodontoid gap and look at the lateral margins of atlas and axis. If atlas is right of

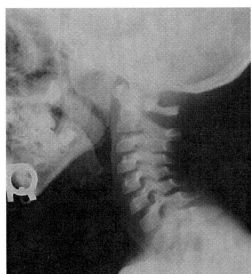

Illustration 18

Lateral cervical x-ray

Note forward cervical curve, distance between C2 spinous and posterior arch of atlas (A) is equal to distance between occiput and posterior arch (B).

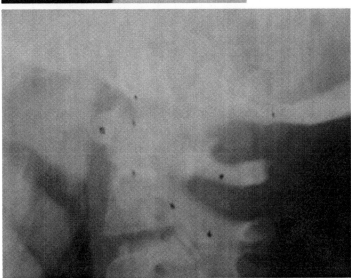

Illustration 19
Lateral x-ray
Enlargement of 18

Dots will be used to draw foramen magnum line, atlas plane line, odontoid line and lamina line of C2.

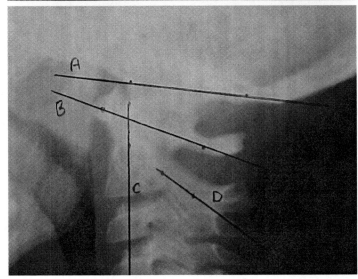

Illustration 20

Lateral x-ray
Lines drawn on 19

A – foramen magnum line
B – atlas plane line
C – odontoid line
D – lamina line of C2

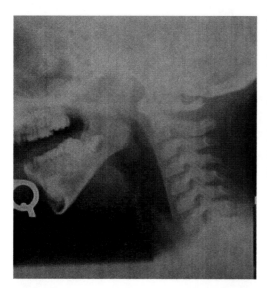

Illustration 21

Lateral cervical x-ray

AI atlas

Note posterior arch approaches occiput. Straightened cervical curve and the anterior tilt of C2 are adaptations to the atlas subluxation.

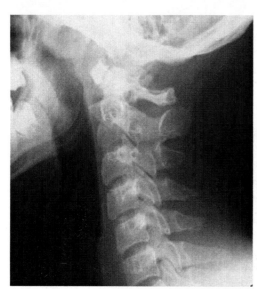

Illustration 22

AS atlas

Posterior arch of atlas approaches spinous of C2. C2/C3 posterior joints are clearly visible indicating rotatory misalignment.

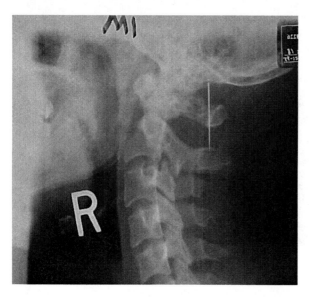

Illustration 23

Lateral cervical x-ray

Posterior C2

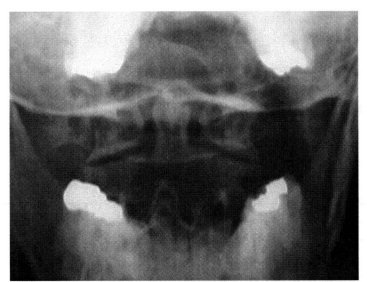

Illustration 24

APOM x-ray
Viewed from posterior.
Illustrations 24, 25, 26 are the same films. C2 appears spinous left of the dens. Illustration 26 shows the dens slightly right of condyle midpoint. C2 has probably moved with atlas.

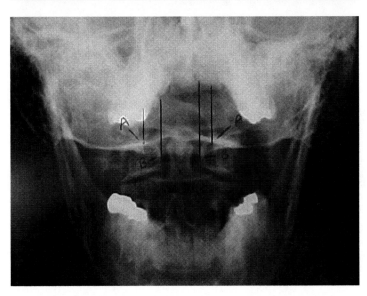

Illustration 25

APOM x-ray
Viewed from posterior

A – Medial inferior tip of condyle
B – Medial aspect of lateral mass

Distance between A and B is larger on left indicating a right misalignment

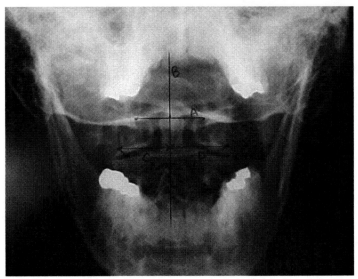

Illustration 26

APOM x-ray
Viewed from posterior
A – line connecting inferior medial tips of condyles
B – line bisecting A and at 90 degrees to A
C and D – distance from B to lateral aspects of lateral masses
D is longer than C indicating right misalignment

axis, the interodontoid gap will be larger on the right and the right inferior lateral margin of atlas will be right of the corresponding point of axis. In this case I would be inclined to adjust atlas.

If axis is right of atlas, then the interodontoid gap will be smaller on the right and you may have found that both the atlas and axis were misaligned right of the condyle midpoint. You now know that both atlas and axis have side slipped right and axis moved further than atlas. In this case, I would be inclined to adjust axis.

Let's overview the APOM analysis. First find the condyle midpoint. Compare atlas to the midpoint. Then compare axis to the midpoint. Last compare axis to atlas.

Remember what we are looking for is how to adjust this person to correct the entire upper cervical misalignment and relieve the interference to the brain stem. If the atlas has sideslipped right you will adjust atlas if it is further right than axis. If the axis is further right than atlas, you will adjust axis. If they have moved together, use patient placement and line of drive to correct them both.

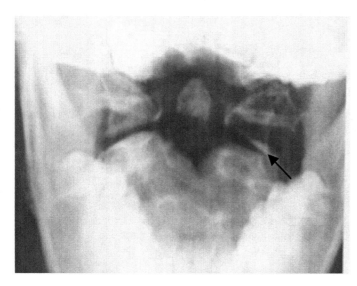

Illustration 27
APOM x-ray
Viewed from posterior

Shadows of teeth are over condyles, left atlas transverse is closer to occiput than right. C2 spinous is quite left of dens. Lateral margin of C1 and C2 do not match on right (see arrow.) C2 body is higher on left.

C1 AL
C2 PLS

Once the basics of x-ray analysis are mastered, the next step is to recognize the malformations and adaptations. Follow the spinal canal and look for a kink or torque. What is the cause of the kink? What is the adaptation?

Adjustment

I remember, when I was a kid, Dad showed me a full spine x-ray. There was a mild scoliosis and he pointed out the misalignment. He said, "Some say you can just beat that spine out like straightening a nail. But you have to remember there is life in that body."

An adjustment is the application of a force that the patient's Innate uses to correct the subluxation. The more precise the force, the better Innate will be able to use it. Although I will write as though the adjustment is a purely mechanical application of force and movement of bones, understand that is not the case.

Once you understand the misalignment, any force that will correct the misalignment and clear the nerve interference is an adjustment. I don't care whether you toggle, use diversified, use an instrument or kick them in the butt. Do what you believe is most likely to clear the subluxation.

Few times will you see an upper cervical misalignment that clearly falls into only one of the misalignment listings. For example, axis may be spinous right and body left and at the same time atlas may be any one of its eight listings. How do you decide what to adjust? Determine what is most likely to correct the entire misalignment and ask Innate!

The first thing I look for is atlas relative to occiput. Then I look at axis relative to atlas. If atlas has misaligned right but the interodontoid gap is larger on the left, then axis has moved farther right than atlas and I might adjust axis with the intention of correcting atlas at the same time. The final decision will be made with confirmation by Innate with a pressure test (explained later.) With proper patient placement, proper segmental contact, and proper line of drive, you will correct even complex misalignments with one adjustment.

An older lady came in one day and went through a list of complaints. Her neck hurt, her back hurt, she had a headache, etc. She had been a patient for a while and I started laughing and said, "I suppose you want all of that to clear up before you leave today."

She smiled as she looked me in the eye and said, "Yes, doctor and I only want one adjustment."

"No adjustment, no results. No results, a mixer was born!"
B. J. Palmer

Toggle Recoil

In my opinion, the toggle recoil is the most precise way to deliver a forceful hand adjustment. It allows for precision and force vectors not afforded by other means. The nail hand is the hand that is touching the patient. The hammer hand is the hand on top of the nail hand. The segmental contact is the point, on the bone, where force is applied

The pisiform is used to make the contact on the spine. If you are adjusting the patient's right side the right hand will be the nail hand and the left hand will be the hammer hand. For left side adjustments reverse hands. The nail hand should be held in a high arch to lock the pisiform in position. (Illustration 28) The pisiform of the hammer hand is then placed in the anatomical snuffbox of the nail hand (Illustration 29) and the fingers of the hammer hand are wrapped around the wrist of the nail hand. (Illustrations 30,31)

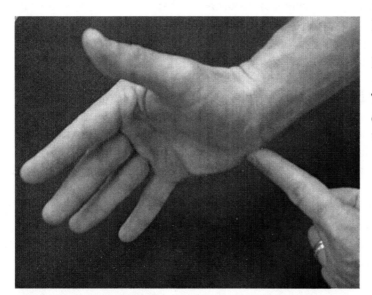

Illustration 28

Demonstration of high arch

The pisiform is used to make contact on the subluxated vertebra.

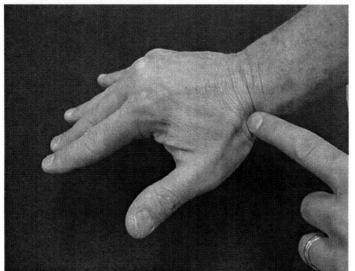

Illustration 29

Anatomical snuffbox

The pisiform of the hammer hand is rolled in here to transfer force through the wrist.

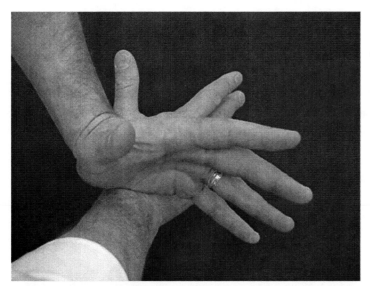

Illustration 30

The pisiform of the hammer hand is being rolled into the anatomical snuffbox of the nail hand.

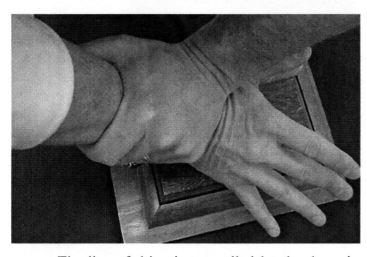

Illustration 31

Hammer hand has now been rolled in, fingers wrapped around the wrist of nail hand, and set up is ready for line of drive.

In this and some of the subsequent views, the set up is on the adjusting trainer.

The line of drive is controlled by the doctor's placement of the episternal notch relative to the pisiform of the nail hand. For example, if the episternal notch is inferior to the nail, the vector of force will include an inferior to superior component. (Illustration 32) Conversely, if the episternal notch is superior to the nail hand the vector of force will include a superior to inferior component. (Illustration 33)

If the episternal notch is posterior to the pisiform, the vector of force will include a posterior to anterior component. (Illustration 34) If the episternal notch is anterior to the pisiform, the vector of force will include an anterior to posterior component. (Illustration 35)

The thrust is a rapid contraction of the arms followed by complete relaxation. Torque can be applied by rotating the arms either clockwise or counterclockwise. For clockwise torque, the right elbow would move toward the body and the left elbow would move away from the body. For counterclockwise torque, the right elbow moves away from the body and the left elbow moves toward the body.

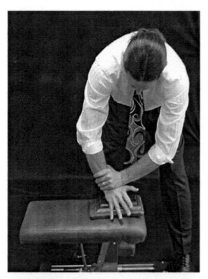

Illustration 32

When the patient is in the knee chest position, the body of the patient will be to the right in the photo and the top of the patient's head will be to the left. The episternal notch (near the knot of my tie) is inferior to the pisiform, in relation to the patient. This placement creates an inferior to superior line of drive or line or correction.

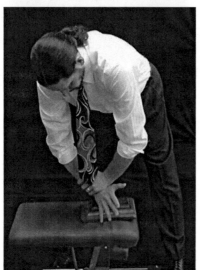

Illustration 33

This illustrates a superior to inferior line of drive. Notice that my tie is hanging superior to my hands.

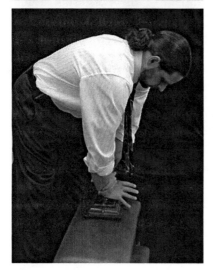

Illustration 34

This illustrates a posterior line of drive. The patient would be facing toward my body. My tie is hanging to the right of my hands and would be posterior in relation to the patient's skull.

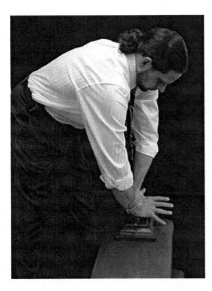

Illustration 35

This illustrates an anterior to posterior line of drive. The patient's face would be turned toward my body.
My tie is to the left or in front of my hands and would be anterior in relation to the patient's skull.

Before attempting to toggle a patient, I recommend time on an adjusting trainer to become proficient. The trainers help improve your speed and control depth of thrust.

Another advantage of the toggle recoil is patient positioning. When adjusting the patient in the side posture position, the patient's spine is neutral, just like when the x-ray was taken. The joints are not in tension. The adjustment corrects the misalignment and puts the joints in their normal relationship.

When using the knee chest position, placement of the head assists the adjustment. If axis is PRS, the patient turns the head to the right. The right turn places tension on the axis to rotate the spinous to the left. However, due to the subluxation, the spinous is right of its normal position and the adjustment aligns the joints reducing, not increasing the tension. The adjustment is not into tension (with the idea of stretching and mobilizing the joint) but releasing tension with the idea of restoring normal alignment.

Interestingly, the head is also turned right to adjust the BR axis. The posterior joints of C2 are misaligned posterior and inferior on C3. When the neck is turned, all posterior joints on the right would normally move posterior and inferior to allow the head to turn. Due to the subluxation, C2 is misaligned and normal movement cannot occur. C2 is already posterior and inferior on C3. Once again the adjustment realigns the joints, moving the joints within the normal range of motion rather than stretching and mobilizing the joint.

> *"...no two torqued subluxations are ever alike in any two people; always varying in degrees.*
> *This means that great care must be used, by Chiropractor, in seeing that his adjustment IS OF THAT CHARACTER AND IS SO DELIVERED THAT IT ACCOMPLISHES THE DIRECTIONS NECESSARY TO CORRECT THE TORQUED SUBLUXATION."*
>
> *B. J. Palmer*

Adjusting Atlas

ASR – The ASR atlas has moved anteriorly and right on the condyles so we want to introduce a force to move it from right to left and from anterior to posterior. Position the patient in the knee chest position with the head turned toward the right. Locate the atlas posterior arch by finding the spinous of C2 and the mastoid process. (Illustration 36) Then come down off of the skull posterior to the mastoid. Place the pisiform of the right hand close to the occiput so that you are superior on the posterior arch. Have your episternal notch superior (toward the patient's head) to the posterior arch. Use clockwise torque. As you adjust, the superior to inferior line of drive created by the position of the episternal notch relative to the pisiform plus the right to left component of the force vector will separate the right lateral mass from the condyle and slide the atlas from right to left. As you torque, move the episternal notch anteriorly and your line of drive will change from superior to anterior correcting the anterior superior components of the misalignment. (Illustration 37)

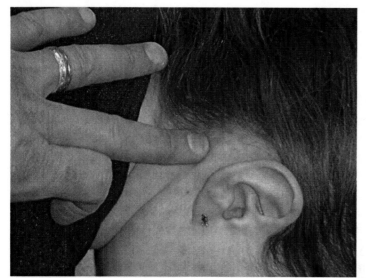

Illustration 36

Finding the segmental contact. The left hand is the hammer hand and is used to find the contact. The pisiform of the right hand is positioned over the palpating finger with the high arch. Complete the set up by rolling in with the hammer hand.

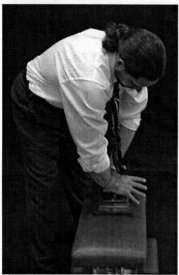 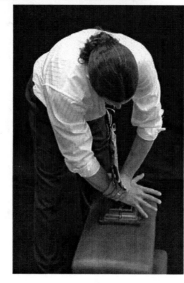

Illustration 37

Left photo demonstrates superior to inferior line of drive at beginning of adjustment. At end of torque, anterior to posterior line of drive is shown in right photo.

Alternative ASR – If the atlas has tracked anterior on the left condyle, it may correct quite nicely by using the condyle as a fulcrum. Have the patient turn the head to the left on the knee chest table. Come under the posterior arch with the episternal notch inferior and anterior to the pisiform. The force will push the atlas against the condyle and slide the atlas posteriorly. (Illustration 38)

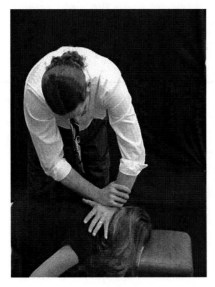

Illustration 38

Alternative ASR adjustment

Inferior to superior line of drive under the posterior arch of atlas on the left side drives the atlas posterior on the left condyle; correcting the anterior (ASR) misalignment.

Clockwise torque can be used to raise the pisiform under the posterior arch and assist in raising the atlas.

ASL – The ASL atlas has moved anteriorly and left on the condyles so we want to introduce a force to move it from left to right and from anterior to posterior. Position the patient in the knee chest position with the head turned to the left. Locate the atlas posterior arch by finding the spinous of C2 and the mastoid process. Then come down off of the skull posterior to the mastoid. Place the pisiform of the left hand close to the occiput so that you are superior on the posterior arch. Have your episternal notch superior (toward the patient's head) relative to the posterior arch. Use counter-clockwise torque. As you adjust, the superior to inferior line of drive created by the position of the episternal notch relative to the pisiform plus the left to right component of the force vector will separate the left lateral mass from the condyle and slide the atlas from left to right. As you torque, move the episternal notch anteriorly and your line of drive changes from superior to anterior correcting the anterior and superior components of the misalignment.

Alternative ASL – If the atlas has tracked anterior on the right condyle, it may correct quite nicely by using the condyle as a fulcrum. Have the patient turn the head to the right on the knee chest table. Come under the posterior arch with the episternal notch very inferior and anterior to the pisiform. The force will push the atlas against the condyle and slide the atlas posteriorly. (Counter-clockwise torque can be used to raise the pisiform under the posterior arch and assist in raising the atlas.)

AIR – The AIR atlas has moved posterior and right on the condyle so we want to introduce a force to move it from right to left and posterior to anterior. Position the patient in the knee chest position with the head turned to the right. Locate the posterior arch by finding the C2 spinous process and the mastoid process then slide down off of the skull posterior to the mastoid. You should now be on the posterior arch right behind the lateral mass. Take contact with the right pisiform. Position the episternal notch superior and posterior. The superior component of the force vector will now separate the right lateral mass from the condyle and the right to left and posterior to anterior components will move the atlas from right to left and posterior to anterior. No torque is needed. (Illustration 39)

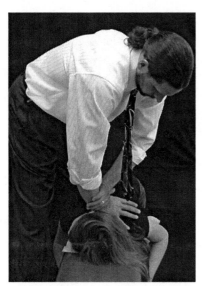

Illustration 39

Correction of AIR

The AIR atlas is corrected with superior to inferior and posterior to anterior line of drive. The segmental contact is the right posterior arch of atlas.

AIL – The AIL atlas has moved posterior and left on the condyles so we want to introduce a force to move it from left to right and posterior to anterior. Position the patient in the knee chest position with the head turned to the left. Locate the posterior arch by finding the C2 spinous process and the mastoid process then sliding down off of the skull posterior to the mastoid. You should now be on the posterior arch right behind the left lateral mass. Take contact with the left pisiform. Position the episternal notch superior and posterior. The superior component of the force vector will now separate the left lateral mass from the condyle and the left to right and posterior to anterior components will move the atlas form left to right and posterior to anterior. No torque is needed.

AS – The AS atlas is tricky to adjust by hand because we are taking contact on a lateral side and always introducing a lateral component in the force vector. However, contact under the posterior arch with a very inferior to superior line of correction (episternal notch toward patient's sacrum) can be used and duplicated on the opposite side if necessary.

AI – For the same reason as the AS this one is also tricky. Contact on the superior portion of the posterior arch with a very superior to inferior and posterior to anterior line of drive can be used and duplicated on the opposite side if necessary.

Note: When palpating the posterior arch, look at the lateral film to determine exact position on the patient.

Adjusting Axis

PRS – The axis PRS has rotated with the axis spinous right of body and right of center of condyles. I use the axis spinous as the segmental contact. Position the patient on the knee chest table with the head turned to the right. Place the right pisiform on the right side of the spinous. Stand so that the episternal notch is anterior and superior to the pisiform. The line of drive is then right to left, anterior to posterior and superior to inferior. This will drive the axis inferior on the right articulation of C3 and the spinous will move toward midline.

PLS – The axis PLS has rotated with the axis spinous left of body and left of center of condyles. Use the axis spinous as the segmental contact. Position the patient on the knee chest table with the head turned to the left. Place the left pisiform on the left side of the spinous. Stand so that the episternal notch is anterior and superior to the pisiform. The line of drive is then left to right, anterior to posterior and superior to inferior. This will drive the axis inferior on the left articulation of C3 and the spinous will move toward midline.

Body right – The axis body has moved to the right relative to the atlas and the spinal canal. The segmental contact is the lamina pedicle junction of C2. Find the axis spinous and the atlas transverse process. Follow the axis lamina from the spinous. The right hand will be the nail hand so place the right pisiform on the lamina pedicle junction of C2. Position the episternal notch inferior to the contact. The inferior to superior component of the force vector will raise the axis on the right and the right to left component will correct the right misalignment.

Body left – The axis body has moved to the left relative to the atlas and the spinal canal. The segmental contact is the lamina pedicle junction of C2. Find the axis spinous and the atlas transverse process. Follow the lamina from the spinous. The left hand will be the nail hand so place the left pisiform on the lamina pedicle junction of C2. Position the episternal notch inferior to the contact. The inferior to superior component of the force vector will raise the axis on the left and the left to right will correct the left misalignment.

Note: During the descriptions of adjusting, I did not mention tissue pull. When you palpate to find the segmental contact point, use the hammer hand. Once the segmental contact has been found, hold the position with your finger and place your pisiform over the finger. Then pull the tissue slightly in the direction of thrust and position the pisiform on the segmental contact of the vertebra.

Part 3: Art

Chiropractic is a philosophy, science and **art**. The art of chiropractic is the knack of doing what we do. The art incorporates the philosophy and science and individualizes chiropractic to the specific chiropractor and patient.

"The Paris doctors give the back bone a general overhauling, very similar to the Osteopaths, whereas I adjust only one vertebra, making the adjustment direct and specific, the difference being that one move adjusts, while the other manipulates, the dissimilarity indicates that one of the methods must be an improvement upon the other."

D. D. Palmer

Consultation

The first thing I want to do is tell the chiropractic story. Every patient is required to read and sign my terms of acceptance. The terms of acceptance defines health, vertebral subluxation, and adjustment. The patient then understands that I have no intention of performing a medical diagnosis, treating symptoms, etc. I then ask the patient what has brought him or her to my office and find out what they are hoping to get from me. I then tell them once again what I do and offer to provide an examination.

I have to admit that I get lazy and forget to keep telling the chiropractic story. I figure if I told them once they ought to get it. After about five years in practice, one of my patients (a former chiropractor) made a sign for me and hung it in the office. The sign said "Subluxations – who needs them? You don't." I was embarrassed by how many of my patients said, "What is a subluxation?" We have to keep telling them.

Sometimes we forget the importance of making sure patients understand the chiropractic story. I met a man socially and he told me he wouldn't be alive if it weren't for chiropractic. He had scoliosis and went in three times a week. His brother was a chiropractor. His wife went to a chiropractor. I thought this guy knew about chiropractic.

After I had known this man for several months he confided that he was losing faith in chiropractic. He would feel better for a while but results just didn't last. I told him about the upper cervical approach and he decided to try it. His first adjustment held and he couldn't believe it when I wouldn't adjust him on the second visit. He still didn't feel any better. I told him to give it time. Pretty soon he was feeling better and he got his wife to come in. She had been in a car wreck and wasn't improving – she started feeling better.

He then told me he wanted to take me to breakfast and talk about helping me promote my practice. At breakfast, he asked me what niche of the market I wanted.

"Do you want rich people, old people, children or what?"

"Bring me sick people," I said.

"What do you mean?"

I told him the chiropractic story. He had never heard it before and had no idea that we took care of sick people. In fact, he called his brother, the chiropractor, and asked him about me because he thought I made the whole thing up. Now here was a man whose brother was a chiropractor and he had been a chiropractic patient for 20 years and he had never heard the chiropractic story. What impact did that have?

A short time later he said, "I've got one for you."

"What have you got?"

"I was baby sitting for some friends and they have a five year old who has never been potty trained. He never knows when he has to go to the bathroom. They've had him checked by all kinds of experts. Do you think you can help him?"

"You know the story – bring him in and let's see."

Two weeks after his first adjustment the little boy felt the urge to go the bathroom for the first time. He was only adjusted a few times. The family moved away but I talked with his mother ten years later and she said he was doing fine and still remembered what chiropractic had done for him. That not only changed his life but the lives of his brothers and sisters who helped clean him up. He was the youngest of five.

All because I told the chiropractic story.

History

The taking of a case history for chiropractic purposes is often overrated. The medical profession stresses the case history to reduce the possible diagnoses from hundreds to a few. They then perform an examination to determine which of the possible diagnoses is most probable.

From a chiropractic standpoint, we start with one question: Is the patient subluxated? Given that the patient is alive; has an Innate Intelligence; has a nervous system, including medulla oblongata/brain stem/spinal cord; has a spine, including occiput, atlas, axis; and has probably been born by being pulled from the birth canal by the head, fallen, and had a car wreck or some other trauma – it is not only possible – it is likely that our patient is subluxated.

The chiropractic examination will tell us whether or not a subluxation exists; without the necessity of the patient's opinions as to what he or she thinks the problem is.

The importance of the case history is not so much to help get the patient well but for legal considerations (for example to document personal injury, employment related injury, other insurance related issues, or referral considerations). Also due to their previous experience, patients often believe that it is important for them to tell us what is wrong. If you wish to indulge and reinforce their beliefs, go ahead – it is easier than changing them. So collect whatever data you feel is appropriate. I do ask patients why they came to see me and I do follow their symptoms – however I do so for fun – because I like to hear the miracles, not because it alters my practice objective or plan of care.

"Today the Chiropractor approaches his case as a problem, desiring to work WITH THIS INNATE INTELLIGENCE IN BODY OF PATIENT THAT INNATE IN PATIENT MIGHT MAKE THE ADJUSTMENT; thereby, ONCE AND FOR ALL, correcting the vertebra to its ABSOLUTE NORMAL position."

B. J. Palmer

Physical Examination

Some chiropractors find it fun to perform a lengthy physical examination on patients, correct the subluxation, then perform a physical examination once again to see what has changed. The danger lies in getting lost in the medical diagnosis (perhaps referring out for worthless and harmful therapies) and failing to provide a good chiropractic examination.

When I was a student I had a retired nurse for a patient. She was quite appalled that I did not wash my hands between patients. I told her I never put my fingers where they didn't belong and she had nothing to worry about. Fortunately, she had a sense of humor and the good sense to know that I was right.

I personally don't care what a patient's blood pressure reads, how much they weigh or how tall they are. In fact, one year as a gag gift I gave my wife a set of bathroom scales for Christmas. When we told one of her friends, the friend said that she was surprised that I didn't have scales at my office. I told her I had never had a patient come in who didn't know he was overweight. Why point out the obvious?

What tests can we perform that will help us decide whether or not this patient is subluxated? I prefer to use skin temperature analysis, leg check, palpation and pressure tests.

"When any chiropractor attempts to practice any phase of medicine he deceives himself and his patient and restrains himself from learning chiropractic and his patient from receiving it and its results."

B. J. Palmer

Skin Temperature Analysis

Skin temperature analysis can be performed using a variety of instruments. I prefer instruments with sensors on each side of the spine so that the right side of a vertebral level is compared to the left side of the same level. This method began with the neurocalometer invented by Dossa Evins.

Single sensor instruments can be used to compare left and right sides (by holding first on one side and then on the other) or to compare levels above and below.

Many instruments are now available using thermocouple sensors (as did the neurocalometer) or infrared sensors. The sensors can be attached to a processor with either a video or paper output.

I use an instrument with bilateral infrared sensors, which gives a printout of the difference between right and left sides up the center and the actual temperature rounded to the nearest degree on each side. I consider a good temperature graph to be balanced from right to left and within one degree from top to bottom with no pattern.

Upper cervical chiropractors use either a break or pattern system of temperature analysis. The break analysis looked for a major temperature difference between left and right sides of the spine at the upper cervical area. The patient was then adjusted and a balance of temperature indicated that the adjustment was successful.

The pattern system looked for the difference between the left and right sides of the spine to be unchanging or in pattern. (Illustration 40) The patient was examined several times. After a pattern was established, the patient was adjusted and a change or breaking of the pattern indicated that the correction was successful. The idea is that a healthy body is constantly adapting to its changing environment and not changing (pattern) is an indication of a loss of health.

Temperature scans can be performed full spine or regionally. If you want to convince yourself of the effect of upper cervical care on the rest of the spine, take full spine graphs. The scans can be taken with the patient seated or prone. In the interest of saving time, I prefer prone. For a full spine scan, I start at the second sacral tubercle and glide the instrument toward the head. Follow the contours of the spine and hold the hair superiorly so that the instrument can measure the temperature over the occiput. Stop the scan at the occiput.

For a cervical scan, start the scan at the inferior tip of C7 spinous and stop on the occiput. Follow the cervical curve and hold the hair up if necessary. Remember that when you test temperature you are using one of the few tests available to check the autonomic nervous system. (Illustration 41)

> *"Bodily temperature above or below normal is pathologic."*
>
> *D. D. Palmer*

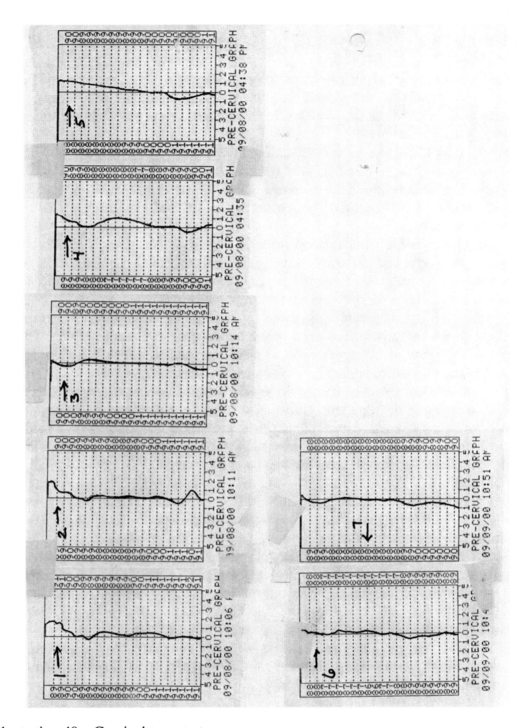

Illustration 40   Cervical temperature scans

The date and time of the exam are given at the bottom. 1 and 2 show a break to the right at the upper cervical area. The scans were taken 5 minutes apart and are quite similar or in pattern. After adjustment the pattern has cleared as shown at 3. Patient returned in the afternoon with a return of the break at 4. It did not clear as well at 5 but I left him alone and checked the next day. The graph the following day shows the break cleared at 6. However, light pressure adjustment warmed the graph up from 86 to 88 (compare the temperatures at 7 with the same area on the chart marked 6.)

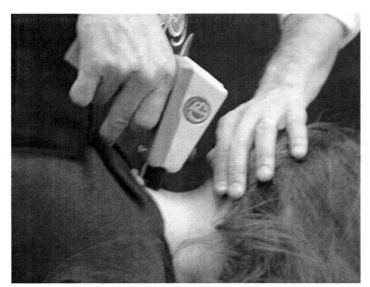

Illustration 41

Taking a cervical scan

First prepare the field by holding the hair and clothing out of the way. Follow the curve of the spine to get an accurate reading.

"Heat regulation is the most important problem which physiologists have to study. When it exists in a normal degree we have health; when there is too much or not enough, we have disease. The body - somewhere and somehow - possesses the ability to control the production of heat and to offset its loss."

D. D. Palmer

Leg Checks

Leg checks can be performed prone or supine. As with any test your consistency and accuracy will determine the value of the test.

For a supine leg check, the patient should be instructed to sit on the end of the table, push herself straight back until her lower legs are well supported on the table, and then lie down on her back. The patient should be helped to recline with support under the neck while holding onto the doctor's arm. Also remember to help the patient get up using the same support procedure. (Illustration 42)

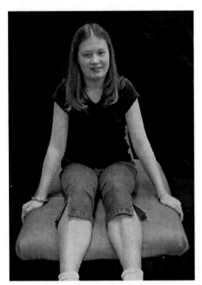 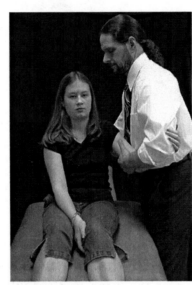

Illustration 42

In the left photo, my daughter, Melissa, demonstrates sliding back on the table. The right photo shows her holding my left arm while I support her head and neck with my right hand.

Once the patient is supine, hold each shoe by the heel with two fingers under the back of the heel, thumbs down side of shoe, and the ring and little fingers under the bottom of the heel. Turn the feet as little as possible yet enough to make the shoes parallel to each other. Then while holding gentle, equal, pressure against both feet, sight down the top border (where the sole meets the upper) of the soles to determine if the legs are balanced. Make sure that you use equal pressure on both feet. The pressure ensures that the shoes are snug against the feet. Sighting down the tops of the soles gives nice even surfaces to compare. (Illustration 43)

A short leg indicates pelvic misalignment (usually caused by vertebral subluxation) or anatomical deficiency. Innate will normally adapt to less than half an inch of anatomical deficiency and show balanced legs when no subluxation is present. I assume that the short leg is caused by subluxation, until proven otherwise.

The best way to perform a leg check prone is to ask the patient to stand on a table that will lower them to horizontal. Simply have the patient stand in the middle of the table and lean onto it. The spine should stay in its usual upright pattern of distortion as you lower the patient.

If you do not have a suitable table, the patient can be asked to center the knees on the end of the table and then lower herself down. (Illustration 44) One problem with leg checks is that the patient can lie down crooked and distort the test. Once the patient is down check her position. Is she centered on the table? Does she appear to be straight? If

©2002 Robert Clyde Affolter

she is not straight, is her posture due to sloppy placement or is it the posture you are trying to measure? If in doubt, get her up and try again.

Once the patient is prone, hold the shoes with the thumbs at the bottom of the heels or just anterior to the heel. The fingers stabilize the foot. Turn the feet as little as possible yet enough to make the shoes parallel. Use gentle even pressure against the bottom of the shoes. Then, using the tops of the soles of the shoes compare the leg length. (Illustration 45)

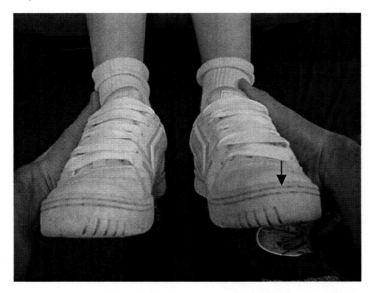

Illustration 43
Supine leg check

Firm (not heavy) pressure against the bottom of the shoes holds the shoes against the feet. Turn the feet so that the soles are parallel and sight down the tops of the soles. The stitching around the tops of the shoes (see arrow) gives a nice mark for comparison.

Also note the condition of the shoes while doing a leg check. One patient came in complaining of sciatica symptoms. During the leg check, I noticed that he had new shoes and one heel was about one eighth inch thicker than the other heel. After adjustment, I showed him his shoes. His back pain coincided with the day he started wearing the shoes on a daily basis. He exchanged the shoes and felt fine.

The leg check should also show a pattern if the patient is subluxated. If the left leg is short and the patient walks around and then the left leg is short again, then you have a pattern, the left leg is short. What is causing the pattern? Is it due to careless, sloppy patient placement? Is it due to careless, sloppy evaluation on the part of the chiropractor? Or is it due to a vertebral subluxation, with resultant nerve interference and muscle imbalance? If the left leg is short the first time and the right leg is short the second time, the test is of no value and you must ask yourself the same questions regarding careless, sloppy examination procedures.

I usually perform the leg check prone. Instruct the patient to get on the table with the knees equal distance from the end of the table then lower the body down using the arms. (Illustration 44) Once again, how the shoes are held will make a big difference in the accuracy of the test. Thumbs under the soles of the shoes apply firm, even pressure and the fingers support the shoes. Turn the feet so that the soles are parallel and sight down the top of the soles. (Illustration 45)

If the patient has a short leg, I continue with the Derifield tests. First I release the feet, then I ask the patient to turn the head to the right and then compare the legs. (Illustration 46) Release the feet and ask the patient to turn the head to the center. Compare the legs again. Release the feet and ask the patient to turn the head to the left. Compare the legs again. If the short leg becomes longer when the head is turned, the cervical syndrome is positive to the side the face is turned. Cervical syndrome is an indication that movement of the cervical spine is having an effect on the musculature of the pelvis and changing the leg length.

Next, I flex the legs at the knees, while watching the leg length. If the short leg becomes the long leg when the legs are flexed, the test is positive and may indicate the need for a pelvic adjustment. (Illustration 47)

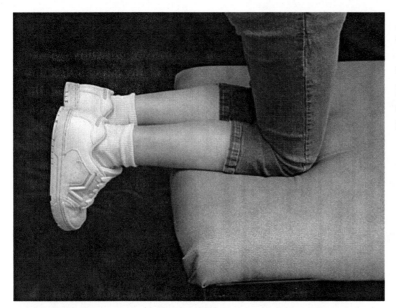

Illustration 44

Getting on the table for a prone leg check. Knees are equal distance from the end of the table.

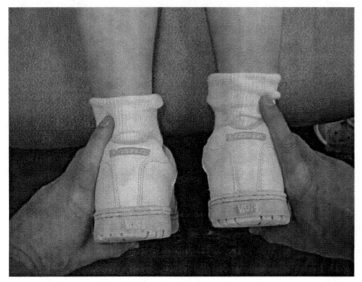

Illustration 45

Prone leg check

The thumbs under the soles and the fingers along the ankles give good control of the feet. The stitching around the shoe gives a sharp line for comparison.

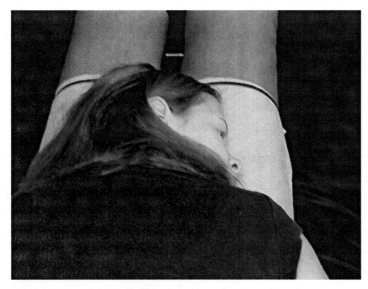

Illustration 46
Modified Derifield
Compare the leg length with the patient's head turned toward the right. Release the legs and have the patient return the face to the center. Compare the legs. Have the patient turn the face to the left. Compare the legs again. A change in leg length, especially a short leg becoming long, indicates a possible cervical subluxation.

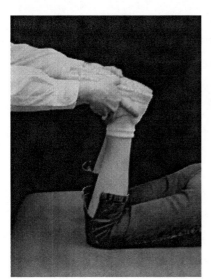

Illustration 47

The final step in the prone leg check is to flex the legs at the knees. The legs must be brought straight up and deviation to the side will invalidate the leg check. As I sight between the feet, I look up the patient's spine and make sure the feet are centered. Then I make the feet parallel and compare the shoes.

"Chiropractic Principles. Nerves heat the body; normal heat is health; heat in a degree more or less than normal is dis-ease. pressure on nerves causes an excess of heat. Metabolism is normal when heat is natural - a condition known as health."

D. D. Palmer

Palpation

Palpation for muscle tension, tissue tone and the position of the bones can also be helpful. Tight neck muscles often accompany a subluxation and the patient will often report some sore or tender spots in the neck.

One way to palpate the upper cervical area is with the patient seated. Place the right third finger on the right mastoid and the left third finger on the left mastoid. Slide the fingers forward and down to find the atlas transverse processes. Does one transverse feel superior to the other, indicating a lateral sideslip to that side? Does one transverse feel anterior or posterior compared to the other?

Now bring your fingers around and find the axis spinous. Does the spinous feel midline to the occiput? Follow the lamina away from the spinous to the lamina pedicle junction. Do the left and right sides feel the same or does one feel posterior to the other?

During the entire palpation process you are also feeling for muscle tightness, tissue tone and asking the patient for areas of tenderness. Areas of tenderness will usually reduce once the subluxation is corrected and give you something else to write down if you are trying to justify care to third party payers. These areas are also often unknown to the patient until you point them out and patients often appreciate knowing that you can find problems that they hadn't even told you.

I personally do not put much emphasis on palpation at this stage of my exam. Too often conclusions reached by palpation are contradicted when the x-rays are developed. What is right – palpation or x-ray? I use the pressure tests described later to help me decide.

By now I have the data to determine whether the patient is subluxated and am ready to report my findings and get the patient's consent for x-rays, if necessary.

"A careful check-up of The PSC spinographic laboratories with my most careful palpation proves 80% of mistakes. Can it be wondered why we do not now and cannot rely upon palpation as being an efficient method?"

B. J. Palmer

Taking X-rays

Next, I will describe a way to take the standard two views of APOM (anterior to posterior open mouth) and neutral lateral. At one point in my career, I was taking neutral lateral, flexion, extension, APOM, lower cervical AP, base posterior, and two diagonals. I have also taken nasiums and stereo films. It is all a matter of how accurate you want to be and how you want to practice. The films I describe are often taken by the average practitioner and can be taken by a cooperative radiologist (if you are willing to train her.)

The true upper cervical specialists use an x-ray chair, precision aligned x-ray frame and head clamps. The patient is often positioned in what the patient believes to be a straight, seated posture with the patient's eyes closed. When a patient closes his eyes and uses his position sense to determine what is straight, the head will often be in flexion or extension, with a right or left tilt. The patient's body is then moved to preserve the neck distortion and make the head centered on the film. If you want to increase your skills I recommend you take classes from doctors skilled in taking upper cervical films.

The order of taking the films makes no difference for my purposes. To take a neutral lateral have the patient stand with a shoulder against the cassette holder and look straight ahead. Make sure the hard palate is slightly elevated.

This is not the neutral lateral usually taken by upper cervical practitioners. It is a modification picked up from Dr. Walter V. Pierce. He wanted to analyze the cervical curve and did not want to wonder if the curve was reversed just because the patient's head was in flexion. With the hard palate slightly elevated, if the patient has a forward curve it will show up. If the most inferior aspect of the nose is above the level of the mastoid, you will probably have good placement.

Place the central ray over the atlas and perpendicular to the film. Open the collimator to get the lower cervicals. Having the central ray over the atlas will produce less distortion at atlas and aid the analysis. If you use 10" x 12" film, you can shoot to the center of the film. If you use 8" x 10" film, you will have to position the center of the film lower than the central ray to get the lower cervicals. (This may be impossible if you have an automatic collimator).

Perform one final check of the patient before taking the film. Look for rotation of the head by comparing the distance from the eyes to the sides of the head. Remove all rotation. Make sure the head is straight by comparing the glabella to the chin and leveling the eyes. Straighten the head. Make sure the hard palate is slightly elevated as described previously. Central ray is over atlas. Film is properly positioned. Right or left marker is on cassette holder. Collimate to film and take the film

To take the APOM, have the patient look straight ahead, facing the tube. Place the central ray perpendicular to the film and through the transverse process of atlas (right under the mastoid). Have the patient open the mouth as wide as possible. If the central ray is in the center of the mouth, you will usually be able to see the atlas and condyles. Have the patient raise or lower the chin as necessary to get the atlas framed by the teeth. You may have to increase your x-ray technique a little to get through the occiput. When done properly you should see the atlas, condyles and axis.

As with the lateral, make sure the head is straight, with no rotation. Double check - central ray to patient and center of film, head straight with no rotation or tilt, right or left marker, collimate to film. Take the film.

Pressure Test

Before I attempt an adjustment I check the patient once again and make sure they are still subluxated and that the pattern is still the same – same short leg and temperature is pattern. Next, I use a pressure test to determine what force is most likely to appeal to Innate.

To perform a pressure test I perform a prone leg check then gently press on the segmental contact in the direction I believe will correct the subluxation. Then I quickly check the legs to see if the short leg balances. If the legs balance, that is an indication that the subluxation is being reduced and I wait for the leg to shorten and then adjust the patient. Remember to wait for the leg to shorten again. If it doesn't shorten, have the patient walk and then perform the leg check again. If the legs are still even, rerun the temperature scan. The pressure test will sometimes prove to be an adjustment.

If the patient's legs are even, the pressure test can be used to test for subluxation by gently tapping on the suspected subluxation (in the direction of correction) and watching for a short leg. If the patient is subluxated the gentle tap will disrupt the adaptations and a leg will be short. If the pressure test is negative I recommend waiting before attempting an adjustment. If the temperature scan is not clear, I look for areas of abnormal energy or tone and use light pressure techniques.

Remember it is important to leave patients alone if they are not subluxated. That cannot be overstressed. Too often we try to accomplish too much. You can't beat someone back to health, so if in doubt, don't.

"Chiropractic is defined as being the science of adjusting by hand any or all luxations of the 300 articular joints of the human body; more especially the 52 articulations of the spinal column, for the purpose of freeing any or all impinged nerves which cause deranged functions. Ninety-five per cent of these are caused by vertebral luxations which impinge nerves."

D. D. Palmer

Light Force Adjustments

Correcting subluxations using sustained light pressure has long been a part of chiropractic. I believe that the only way to effectively learn this procedure is through hands-on workshops. However, it is appropriate to discuss my hypothesis concerning this approach.

From a standpoint of physics, our bodies are patterns of electromagnetic energy. Therefore, when we palpate, we are palpating energy fields. For example, if you press on a solid wood 2 x 4 stud, you are feeling the energy field of the wood. The wood (and the energy field) feels strong and firm. If you press on an older, decaying stud you will feel it give under your fingers. The energy field is weak.

Similarly, when you palpate patients, some will feel very strong (for example the muscular weight lifter) and some will feel weak (a baby.) Surprisingly, if you very carefully and lightly palpate along the spine of the weight lifter you will probably find areas that feel more like the baby. Those areas of weakness or loss of tone are a result of a weakness in the energy field, an area of dissonance (or simply a spot.)

The areas of weakness are due to lack of energy through the nervous system. The reasons a subluxation doesn't automatically correct itself are because of osseous locking, ligament blockage (e.g. nucleus pulposus off center), or *because of nerve interference to the muscles of the subluxated vertebra.* If we supply the correct stimulus to the muscles, the subluxation will self correct.

Once the spot is found, light pressure can be applied to correct the subluxation and bring the area into resonance. The depth and direction of pressure is determined by following the feeling of dissonance and matching the body. Too light pressure will have no effect and too heavy pressure will produce resistance in the body. Light pressure adjusting has become one of my favored adjusting procedures because to do it right you must work with Innate and if you do it wrong Innate can easily resist.

Start at occiput and palpate between the occiput and atlas. Start midline and palpate both sides as far anterior as the atlas transverses. Work your way down both sides of the neck over the transverses and midline over the spinouses. Then lightly pass your hand down the rest of the spine, over the sacroiliac joints and to the coccyx.

Treat light pressure adjustments just as seriously as toggle recoil. Post check with leg checks and temperature scan and make sure an adjustment has been made. I find that once pressure tests and leg length tests are negative I can clear a graph with light pressure adjustments only. In fact, many times light pressure adjustments are all that is ever required.

> *"Dr. Arnold and I agree, in that skill in adjusting is shown by the ability of the adjuster to move vertebrae with the least force or pressure possible. She gives 'pressure rather than thrust.' I give thrust rather than pressure; that is, I find that the quicker the same amount of force or pressure is given, the more effectual is the result. I desire to move vertebrae with as little force as possible."*
> *D. D. Palmer*

Post Adjustment

For twelve years, I rested patients for at least ten minutes after every adjustment. I had rest booths with recliners or rest tables where the patient could stay until it was time for their post examination. Then I would do the leg check and temperature scan and look for a break in pattern. Although I no longer use rest booths, I still do post adjustment examination on every patient. I expect the legs to be balanced and the temperatures to be more balanced or warmer or hopefully both.

Whether you decide to install rest areas or not is up to you. The point is to give Innate time to make changes after the adjustment. If you do a temperature scan immediately after an adjustment you may see huge temperature difference. However, patience will often show that the adjustment was indeed made. If you react too quickly you will be interfering in Innate's corrective process and delay the healing.

On the other hand, I know some chiropractors site the above example and state that as their reason for never doing a post examination. If you check a patient every day, and most of your patients do not need an adjustment on the second day, then I salute you. You are doing a fine job. However, if you do not perform a post adjustment examination, and you are adjusting patients every time they come in – then how do you know you ever really adjusted them?

I attended a seminar put on by a Blair practitioner. He never performed a post adjustment examination, but claimed superiority over general practitioners because he does less adjusting. Monday morning a patient asked what I did over the weekend. When I told her I attended a seminar, she asked how the instructor practiced. As it happened, her former chiropractor was a Blair practitioner. I told her that he practices just like your last chiropractor.

She said, "So he is somewhere between a general manipulator and you."

"I think he would be quite upset if I told him that," I replied.

"Well it's true. The first guy I went to just went crunch, crunch, crunch down my spine and maybe he would get it and maybe he wouldn't. I often felt worse after adjustment. The second chiropractor was better, he would run the instrument up my neck and do a leg check before he adjusted me, but he never did it after adjustment. So maybe he would get it and maybe he wouldn't. I often felt worse. You always check me after you adjust me and I have never left feeling worse. I may not feel any better but I don't feel any worse."

A post adjustment examination elevates us just a little more and improves the odds by knowing when nerve interference has been corrected. I always perform a post adjustment examination. If examination proves that nothing happened, I rethink and try again. If the examination shows a wonderful clear out, I collect my fee and schedule another checkup. If the examination is questionable, I will usually rest the patient a little longer and then re-examine. If still questionable, I schedule another checkup and give Innate more time.

I believe it is the examination – adjustment – post examination that makes chiropractic a science. Once while testifying on a personal injury case, an attorney asked me if it was true that the patient was also taking an anti-depressant medication and that it was the medication that made him feel better and not the adjustments. I replied that while I knew nothing about the medication, the patient would come in complaining of pain and my examination showed that he needed an adjustment. I adjusted him and had him rest. He then checked better and felt better with no medication being taken. That indicated to me that it was the subluxation that was causing his pain and the adjustment was helping. Sometimes following symptoms is helpful.

"Away back, when I was a youngster, I made a vow that I would so utilize my life as to be able to leave behind a specific – not for the cure of any and all dis-ease, but that I would leave behind the specific for the CAUSE of ALL DIS-EASE. I have dedicated and consecrated my life to that goal."
B. J. Palmer

Plan of Care

What is your plan of care? The medical doctor examines a patient, prescribes a medication, and then, follows up in two weeks with another examination. The physical therapist practices similarly. When insurance companies began paying chiropractors they expected to see a similar procedure. Rather than practice scientifically and explain chiropractic, many chiropractors simply adopted the physical therapy plan. They prescribe a plan of care with a certain number of weeks duration and two or three manipulations per week and re-examine.

My plan is always the same. I examine the patient on every visit and adjust the subluxation as needed. I often start with daily examinations and then taper off as the patient begins to hold. For example, patients usually begin care with a short leg and by the second or third visit the legs are balanced on the pre-check. That is an indication that they are improving. If the legs are balanced but the temperature scan is pattern, I do a pressure test to check for subluxation and adjust if needed. If the legs are balanced and there is no temperature pattern twice in a row, I reduce the frequency of care. Why continue to see someone daily if they don't need an adjustment? On the other hand if you are adjusting someone three times per week for three weeks and suddenly you reduce the frequency to twice per week, what was your justification?

I continue to check the patient until they are holding the adjustment and the condition is resolved. I then explain the importance of periodic checkups and let the patient decide whether they want health care or symptomatic care.

"The vertebral SUBLUXATION was not new. They were PROduced and Reduced by clashing of INTERNAL with EXTERNAL ACCIDENTAL concussions of forces. These existed from the beginning of time. An ACCIDENT occurred, a vertebral subluxation was PROduced, man got sick. Another subsequent ACCIDENT occurred, a vertebral subluxation was REduced, man got well. D. D. Palmer knew this. What HE did was to take it out of the realms of the ACCIDENTAL FIELD and put the doing into AN INTENTIONAL FIELD, where the ACCIDENTAL FIELD failed and could not overcome itself."
B. J. Palmer

Is The Patient Improving?

How do you answer that question? The patient wants to know. The insurance company wants to know. What do you report?

Some use the need to know as an excuse for doing a medical orthopedic and neurologic examination – they think the insurance company wants to know about positive reflexes and foraminal compression tests. I find they don't care. They just want to know what we are doing and that there is a positive outcome. Patients are the same story. They want to feel better and they want some confidence that you know what you are doing and that your approach is working.

The following is a typical case in my practice. The patient initially presents with a short leg, cervical temperature pattern, possibly a right or left cervical syndrome, possibly positive pelvic Derifield, and the pressure test is positive at the site of subluxation. The patient leaves the office after the first adjustment with an improved temperature scan and legs balanced.

By the third visit, the patient presents with balanced legs but the temperatures may still be pattern. Improvement! If the legs are balanced to begin, then the cervical syndrome and Derifield are automatically not performed and are negative. I then pressure test the area of subluxation and will often get a short leg. I then adjust as indicated by the pressure test. The patient leaves with balanced legs, improved temperatures and negative pressure tests.

Soon the patient presents with balanced legs, temperatures are pattern and the pressure tests are negative. More improvement! I then use the procedure mentioned in light force techniques to improve the temperatures. Finally, the patient presents with legs balanced, temperatures clear, pressure tests are negative and tissue tone is normal. The goal has been reached and no adjustment is given. Now we simply check the patient to make sure the subluxation stays corrected.

All of the foregoing signs of improvement are directly related to the subluxation and have been performed on every visit. I have no problem with performing a posture analysis and range of motion tests on a periodic basis (or any other exam for that matter) but once again let us not make posture or range of motion our practice objective.

In addition to the above, I look for changes on x-rays. I look for motion to improve, cervical curves to be restored, and misalignments to be corrected. X-rays combined with physical findings give an excellent, chiropractic determination of how the patient is progressing. Although some are teaching techniques with a practice objective of restoring the cervical curve or straightening the spine, those are orthopedic (ortho – straight, pedic – pertaining to children) goals. Unless and until straightening the spine and restoring the cervical curve are proven to relieve nerve interference, those are not chiropractic objectives. However, a straightening of the spine or the restoration of the cervical curve often results from correction of a subluxation. Thus proving the loss of cervical curve and scoliosis to be adaptations to the subluxation.

Difficult Cases

If I find I am adjusting the same subluxation in the same manner three consecutive visits, time to rethink. Perhaps I can appeal to Innate in a different manner.

If I have been using toggle, I try light force. If I am having trouble finding spots, I try palpating the patient sitting up, standing up, and prone. I also palpate for spots while the spine is in motion.

I also change my toggle. If I have been using a knee chest position, I try side posture. Try something creative. Once I know the direction of misalignment, there are many force vectors that might help make the adjustment. I pressure test for different vectors and see which vector Innate wants me to use.

I also look at the x-rays again. Is it possible that the atlas I thought was AS is really an AI with a loss of the cervical curve and an occiput in flexion? Is it possible axis is the major instead of atlas? Do I have that hellish situation where atlas is left and axis is right? I re-evaluate the graphs. Am I sure of the pattern? Am I clearing the pattern?

I have also sent patients to a colleague who uses a different technique. That is one of the reasons I have changed techniques. I have taken patients to someone who used a different approach and when it worked I learned the technique.

Our patients deserve the best chiropractic has to offer.

> *"I believe that every Chiropractor thinks that he is specific in his or her adjusting. There are those who adjust every vertebrae for any and every disease; others who adjust every other one on the first day and the alternate ones on the next, thus, in the two days, they surely do not miss any; and still others who adjust any vertebrae which seems to be out of line. They all think they are specific."*
> *D. D. Palmer*

Practice Management

There are many practice management specialists to help you make your practice financially successful. You can be the greatest chiropractor in the world but if you don't make money you won't be able to help many people.

This book has not been about making money. It has been about improving your odds of getting sick people well. I believe that you can have a principled, scientific chiropractic practice based on cash or insurance. In fact, the more you use technology to prove that the person was subluxated and that you corrected the subluxation the fewer problems you will have with insurance.

However, we must also understand that insurance is about spreading risk. Insurance is not about staying healthy. There is no risk to staying healthy. If insurance companies intend to sell policies by telling people that it is health insurance, then insurance companies should have to pay for well checkups.

If the insurance companies revert back to the idea of simply spreading risk of getting sick, then people will have to pay for well checkups with cash. However, our challenge is to show that those who pay for well checkups should get lower premiums because they are healthier. That could be one of the goals of our research endeavors. Find out if patients who are on regular checkup schedules stay healthier than people who don't.

I think you will find there are two primary keys to practice management. One is marketing. People have to know where you are and what you do. You have to be able to get new patients into your office. I have not attempted to cover marketing.

The second key is knowing what to do after they come in. Do you have a logical explanation of chiropractic? Can you explain the importance of a vertebral subluxation? The answers to those questions can be found in the philosophy section of this book. Some practice managers can help you explain what we do. The last part is knowing how to deliver the goods, finding and adjusting a subluxation. Once you have mastered the art of chiropractic, practice managers can help you become more efficient.

The point of this chapter is that this is not a book about being financially successful. I have nothing against making money nor do I have anything against any of the coaches who will help you build your business. I do encourage you to make chiropractic scientific and talk about regular checkups rather than regular adjustments. When you use leg checks and instrumentation and properly explain the findings to your patients, they will come in and ask you how they are doing.

One of my favorite stories is about my son Matt. He was running a fever when he was about three years old. I took him to my office for a checkup. I ran a scan up his neck and looked at the graph. He looked up at me with bright red cheeks and blurry eyes and asked, "Daddy am I sick?"

Imagine a world where everyone understood chiropractic like my three year old. They would come in for a checkup and even if they felt like hell would ask us if they are sick. It all starts with us. Can you look at a little boy with a fever and a clear graph and balanced legs and say, "Nah, you're not sick, you just don't feel good. You'll be okay."

Part 3: Techniques

Is your practice of chiropractic changing? In this part, I present my chiropractic history. I will review some of the techniques that have had the most influence on me and why I changed.

"Let me talk to a practicing Chiropractor, and I'll date his subluxation and its physical and mental interference that produced his standing-still year."

B. J. Palmer

Palmer Upper Cervical Technique

By second quarter at Palmer College, I was attending the Upper Cervical Society and reading B. J. Palmer's green books. My father used toggle recoil and had taught me on his "Thompson Trainer." After investigating the upper cervical approach, I determined to make that the basis of my practice.

I can think of no better place to thank two of my mentors, followers of B. J. Palmer, and strict upper cervical practitioners. When I was an upper quarter student, I was fortunate to intern in the private practice of Dr. E. L. Crowder. As an intern, I got to see chiropractic practiced as a science. New interns had to be able to duplicate the leg checks and instrumentation of experienced interns. In addition, Dr. Crowder took a few hours on weekends to teach chiropractic philosophy. When I decided to locate in Washington State, Dr. Crowder advised me to call Dr. Arthur Thompson.

While I waited for my state exam results, I went to Dr. Thompson's office, one day a week. He let me graph his patients, taught me to read stereo x-rays (which lead to development of three dimensional vision, something I had never had), and introduced me to solid headpiece toggle adjusting. In addition, he looked at x-rays and gave me advice on my "difficult cases" the first few months of my practice. These two chiropractors have had a great influence on my life. Thank you both.

A great thing about upper cervical chiropractic is that you cannot be focused on a condition. It helps break you of that mentality. If someone comes in with a pain in the foot, you look for an atlas/axis subluxation.

I was lucky to have just such a case while still a student. I pressed on the bottom of the patient's foot and she nearly levitated from the table in pain. I x-rayed her and adjusted her atlas. On her next visit I asked how her foot was doing and she said "fine" like nothing was wrong and she had forgotten all about it. I asked her when it got better and she replied, "As soon as you adjusted me."

One of the best books on upper cervical chiropractic is B. J. Palmer's, The Subluxation Specific – The Adjustment Specific (also known simply as Volume XVIII) published by Palmer School of Chiropractic (1934). The book talks about the neurocalometer for determining when to adjust, describes the toggle recoil, and x-ray analysis. However, Volume XVIII was not the end of upper cervical research.

By 1958, the B. J. Palmer Chiropractic Clinic had been in existence for 23 years and seen over 9000 cases of all ages and types of conditions. Over one and a quarter million dollars had been spent on laboratory research equipment and over a million dollars in intangible research. The clinic was divided into two divisions, chiropractic and medical. The medical equipment was the best available and doctors were hired to establish the diagnosis of the patient and determine whether the findings duplicated the previous physician. No medical treatment was provided.

The chiropractic division was built to determine the most effective approach to adjusting patients. New x-ray views were designed to better visualize the misalignment. Base posterior, nasium (Illustrations 48, 49) and diagonal films were researched. The base posterior film is taken by placing the x-ray tube near the patient's knees and shooting through the skull at about a 45 degree angle. The film gives a view of the foramen magnum and atlas. It is typically used to measure rotation of atlas relative to the skull. The nasium film is shot down the atlas plane line and is used to view the atlas relationship to the condyles. The diagonal or oblique views are taken similar to the nasium, but with the patient turned and give another view of the condyle relative to the lateral mass.

Stereo views were used to give a three dimensional view of the spine. To obtain stereo views, the patient is put in head clamps and two films are taken. The first film is taken with left shift of the x-ray tube. The second film is taken with right shift of the tube. The shift distorts the image on the film. The films are then read in a stereo view box, which consists of two view boxes mounted opposing each other. (Illustration 50) One film is placed in the right and the other is placed in the left view box. The films are then viewed by looking in mirrors mounted between the two view boxes. With one film viewed by each eye, the mind fuses the two views and gives the illusion of three dimensions.

Dr. Palmer also built the electroencephaloneuromentimpograph - a prototype of the modern day EEG. He researched the electrical activity from the brain down the spine to determine what was happening to the nervous system.

Above are just a few examples of the research which was done under the direction of Dr. B. J. Palmer, the developer of chiropractic. Few of today's chiropractors are aware of those research efforts. Therefore, they attend seminars taught by "chiropractors" covering medical research on the spine and attempting to apply that research to chiropractic. Two problems arise: First, it is extremely difficult to apply medical research with a chiropractic mindset. The second problem is that we are never made aware of our scientific heritage. This book is a small effort to correct those problems.

"The ONE FINAL AND LAST WORD in the use of any technic is: DOES IT INCREASE OR DECREASE QUANTITY FLOW of mental impulse nerve force, impeded and obstructed by a vertebral subluxation, with the use of this or that technic?"

B. J. Palmer

Grostic Technique

Dr. John D. Grostic, son of the developer of the Grostic Technique, was on faculty at Palmer when I was a student. He had a great sense of humor and I enjoyed having him as a teacher.

The Grostic Technique is the basis of many of the upper cervical approaches including NUCCA and Atlas Orthogonal. The technique uses supine leg check and cervical instrumentation to determine when a subluxation exists. X-rays are analyzed using nasium and base posterior views. The idea is that the atlas should be at right angles to the central skull line on both nasium and base posterior views. (Illustration 48, 49)

Measurements are taken from the films and a formula is derived for a specific, vectored adjustment using a modified toggle. Post x-rays are then taken to determine the efficacy of the adjustment and the vector of adjustment is modified if needed.

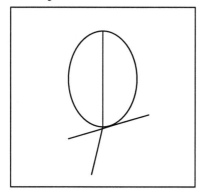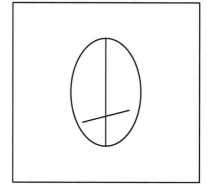

Illustration 48

The diagram on the left represents a nasium x-ray. The oval represents the skull and the center line represents the central skull line. The horizontal line represents the atlas plane line. The lower diagonal line represents the relationship of the lower cervical spine to the atlas. The diagram on the right represents a base posterior film. The vertical line represents the center of the skull. The diagonal line represents the rotation of atlas and is drawn through the center of the atlas transverse foramen. The angles are measured and used to determine a precision adjustment. Post x-rays after the adjustment are used to determine if correction was accomplished and to change the adjustment vector if necessary.

I have heard chiropractors say, "x-rays don't change" and "x-rays change all the time." Both comments are by chiropractors who have not practiced specific x-ray placement and accurate analysis. Attend an Atlas Orthogonal, NUCCA or Grostic seminar and you will get a whole new appreciation for the science of chiropractic.

The first three years of my practice I practiced strictly upper cervical chiropractic. One Friday I had an elderly patient come in complaining of heart problems. Her medical doctor had given her an EKG because she was having weakness and shortness of breath after mild exertion. I couldn't find an upper cervical subluxation but was finding a thoracic subluxation, so I x-rayed her thoracics. I found a mild scoliosis and a suspected subluxation.

Examination proved the thoracic misalignment was a subluxation and I used a Gonstead style adjustment. I told her the adjustment might have an effect on her heart and we scheduled an appointment for Monday.

She came in Monday afternoon and said, "Boy, is my doctor mad at me."

"How come?"

"Well I went in and he had the results of my EKG and told me I needed a whole fist full of pills. I told him I don't either I am fine."

I said, "I didn't tell you to say that!"

"No but I am. Ever since you adjusted me I have felt fine."

That person had been a patient for several years and I wondered if I had missed that thoracic – so I began full spine x-ray of everyone.

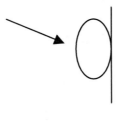 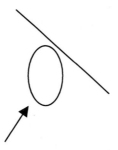

Illustration 49

The ovals represent the skull, the straight lines represent the film holder, and the arrows represent the angle of the x-ray tube. The left diagram is taking a nasium x-ray and the right is taking a base posterior.

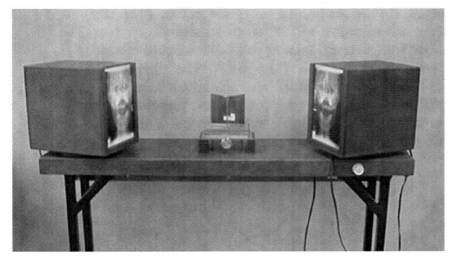

Illustration 50

Stereo view box

The films are analyzed by rotating the view boxes to face each other and looking in the mirrors.

Gonstead Technique

When I was about 12 my family took a vacation to Mt. Horeb, Wisconsin while Dad spent a week with Dr. Clarence S. Gonstead. Dad then began taking full spine x-rays on all patients.

Once again, I was about to follow in his footsteps. I began taking full spine films on all patients but continued taking the upper cervical films as well. Since the Gonstead methodology was part of the curriculum at Palmer, I naturally used that x-ray analysis.

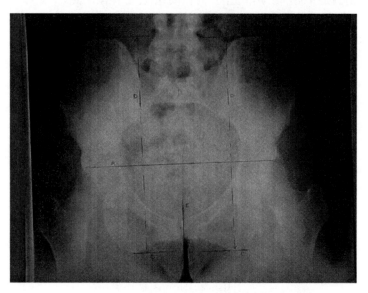

Illustration 51
The Gonstead pelvis analysis

All measurements are relative to the femur head line, drawn across the top of the femur heads. Due to the normal tilt of the pelvis, when one side misaligns posterior and inferior it will show up as longer on the film. The iliums are measured from the most inferior point on the ischial tuberosity to the most superior point on the iliac crest. The longer side is posterior/inferior (PI) and the shorter side is anterior/superior (AS.) Rotation of the ilium is determined by drawing a line perpendicular to the femur head line at the level of the pubic symphysis and aligned with the second sacral tubercle. The line is on the ilium that has rotated external (EX) and the opposite side is internal (IN.)

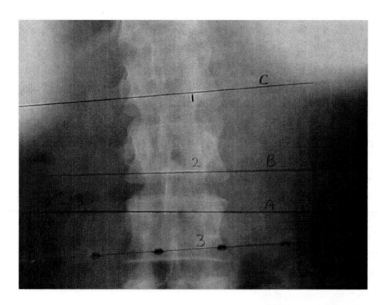

Illustration 52
The Gonstead disc analysis

Lines are drawn representing the end plates of the vertebrae. Parallel lines indicate the nucleus pulposus is centered. Lines A and B are nearly parallel. Lines B and C form a wedge, which is open on the right. The nucleus is off to the right. Spinouses are all PL. The listing is PLI.

The strengths of the Gonstead Technique are the specificity of the adjustments and the examination of the patient. Full spine instrumentation, and motion palpation are performed on every visit and correlated with x-ray to determine when and where to adjust. I have seen many chiropractors claim to be followers of Dr. Gonstead and yet they did not run a nervo-scope (similar to the neurocalometer described previously) on every visit, nor compare motion palpation findings to the x-rays. If you don't do the full examination, how can you get the same results?

Another plus for the Gonstead Technique is the listing system describing misalignment. The right ilium is compared to the left and listed by comparing the posterior superior iliac spine (PSIS) to the opposite side. The listings can be posterior and inferior (PI) or anterior and superior. (AS) The ilium can also rotate with the PSIS going away from the sacrum – external rotation (EX) or toward the sacrum – internal rotation. (IN) (Illustration 51)

When listing vertebral misalignment, only posterior movement is considered, so the first letter of the listing is always P. The spinous is listed as left or right of body and superior or inferior according to the disc wedge on the side of spinous rotation. For example, if the spinous is left of body and the disc is open on the left the listing is PLS. If the spinous is left of body and the disc wedge is closed on the left the listing is PLI. (Illustration 52)

The weaknesses of the Gonstead system are that it is a bottom-up approach. I also prefer to look at the occiput-atlas-axis area as a unit with the idea of correcting all three rather than relating atlas to axis and occiput to atlas. However, the careful approach to examination and the specificity of the adjustments make this technique a nice addition to your practice if you find you need a forceful full spine technique. Before I use a Gonstead style adjustment, I make sure I have a positive pressure test.

Pierce Technique

Drs. Walter Vernon Pierce and Glenn Stillwagon were teaching seminars together and their approach (Pierce Stillwagon Technique – PST) was being taught at Palmer College as an extracurricular course. I completed the course in 1983. Dr. Pierce came and talked to the class and I attended his seminar. After graduation, I attended another seminar. I have never met Dr. Stillwagon so I will only describe my experience with Pierce's work.

A common denominator among all the great chiropractors is chiropractic dedication and conviction. Upper cervical toggle recoil was a big part of PST. The upper cervical approach is seen in the use of instrumentation and x-ray. PST was noted for the double AS and double PI pelvis (Illustrations 53, 54) adjustments. Dr. Pierce may be best known for his work with videofluoroscopy, the fifth cervical adjustment to restore the cervical curve and the flexion and extension lock analysis (Illustration 55.)

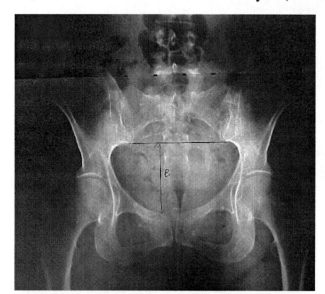

Illustration 53

Double PI pelvis

Increased height of the obturator foramen and the decreased height of the pelvic opening are hallmarks of the Double PI pelvis. Compare to Double AS below.

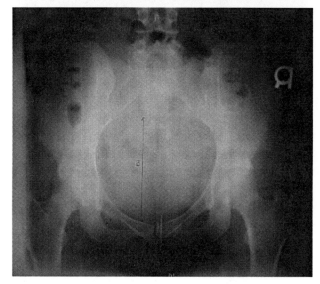

Illustration 54

Double AS pelvis

Increased height of the pelvic opening and decreased height of the obturator foramen are signs of the Double AS pelvis. Compare to Double PI above.

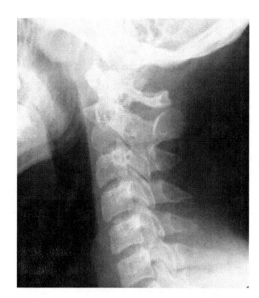

Illustration 55

These are all films of the same patient. The film to the left is a neutral lateral. Notice that the atlas is nearly touching the spinous of C2. The middle films are flexion (on the left) and extension (on the right.) In flexion, the atlas posterior arch barely moves away from axis. In extension, occiput is not moving back on atlas. The listing would be occiput locked in extension. Atlas locked in flexion. The bottom films are flexion and extension taken one hour post atlas adjustment. Compare the movement of occiput and atlas.

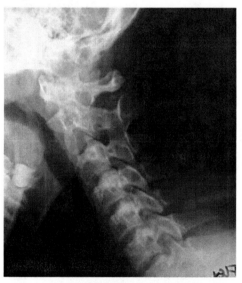

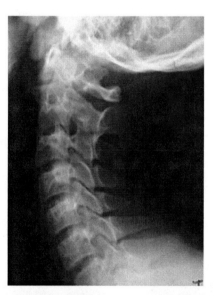

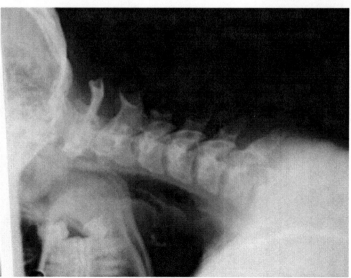

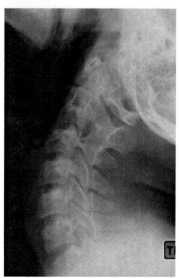

Dr. Pierce put together several different approaches to develop his technique. One of them was Logan Basic and since Logan Basic was also being taught as an extra-curricular class at Palmer, I completed that in 1983. Pierce and Logan were my early experiences with low force adjusting. It was often stated that the force should be less than the pressure one could comfortably stand on the eyeball.

He was constantly using new technology. I bought one of the first Decade IIIR infrared recording instruments that he promoted. It had a single sensor infrared pickup and was used along the full spine. Dr. Pierce is also known for his use of videofluoroscopy to determine vertebral motion, development of the 3-D drop head piece, utilization of the Precision Spinal Adjuster and later a computerized adjusting instrument. The adjusting instruments come with a dual prong attachment for adjusting both sides of atlas simultaneously. (Illustration 56)

One of my patients was losing energy and feared he was dying. I took him to a chiropractor, who was using a videofluoroscopy unit and Precision Spinal Adjuster. Based on our findings, we adjusted atlas, C3 and C5. Within a short time the patient had improved. I bought a table with the 3-D headpiece and a Precision Spinal Adjuster from Dr. Pierce and began doing static flexion and extension films on everyone.

The technique is heavily dependent on either the computerized adjusting instruments or videofluoroscopy to determine the adjustment. I prefer the pressure test and the temperature scans. I always felt there was a weakness in the specificity of the upper cervical approach of Dr. Pierce. Indeed, the more he researched, the more he wound up back to adjusting atlas.

One day a colleague told me about the Blair Technique of matching the atlas to the condyles. The idea made sense so I took the four Blair Technique seminars.

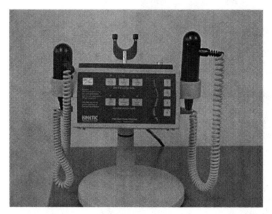

Illustration 56

An early version of the Precision Spinal Adjuster

The dual prong attachment can be seen on top of the instrument.

Blair Technique

Dr. Weldon Muncy was teaching the Blair seminars when I went through them. Now there are several certified instructors teaching the Blair method. The technique is an upper cervical approach using instrumentation (pattern analysis) and leg checks to determine when to adjust and x-ray analysis to create a vectored adjustment.

In contrast to Dr. Grostic who thought the atlas should be perpendicular to the skull, Dr. Blair's research showed that malformation or anomaly was the norm and therefore line drawing analysis was not valid. However, even if malformation exists, Innate will still build the right condyle to match the right lateral mass and the left condyle to match the left lateral mass.

Dr. Blair devised a way to determine if the joint surfaces of atlas were aligned with the condyles. First, take a base posterior film with lead pointers in the ear canals. The film is analyzed by outlining the shape of the condyles on the film. Then each condyle is bisected along its long axis and a line is drawn between the shadows of the lead pointers on the film. The angle formed by the lead pointer line and the line through the condyle tells how much the condyle converges. A film is then taken of each condyle using a Blair head clamp that has ear pointers and a built-in protractor.

Each film is looking exactly down the articulation of the condyle and atlas. If the outside border of the atlas matches the outside border of the condyle there is no misalignment. If the atlas sticks out farther than the occiput, then the atlas is misaligned to the side of the overlap. If the atlas sticks out less than the condyle, then the atlas is misaligned opposite the side of the underlap.

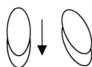

Illustration 57

Diagrams of atlas tracking on the condyle – top of the page is anterior.

Lower ovals represent the lateral masses of atlas. Upper ovals represent condyles of occiput. The two sides are asymmetrical. The left condyle/lateral mass joint has an angle of convergence of zero degrees for ease of demonstration. On the top diagram the atlas has tracked forward on the left condyle and the right condyle shows an overlap (ASR) of atlas (bottom oval) on the condyle. The bottom diagram shows atlas tracking posterior on the left condyle and the right condyle shows an underlap (PIL) of atlas (bottom oval) on the condyle.

In addition to the special protracto views of atlas, Blair practitioners also take stereo lateral views to analyze the alignment of the posterior joints of C2 to C4. (Illustration 58) The posterior joints can misalign posterior and inferior or anterior and superior on either the right or left. The adjustment is designed to match the joint surfaces on the subluxated articulation.

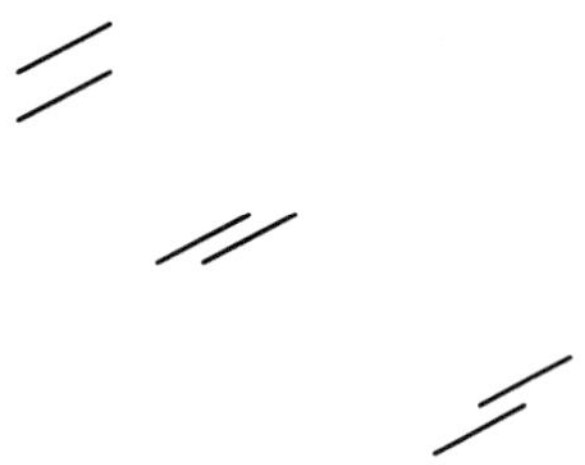

Illustration 58
Misalignment of the lower cervicals. The joint surfaces should match. The Blair oblique lateral is taken with the patient slightly turned so that both left and right posterior articulations are visible. These three diagrams demonstrate alignment, posterior and inferior misalignment, and anterior and superior misalignment.

The Blair adjustment is a toggle, which is vectored to match the shape of the patient's articulations.

I bought the Blair head clamp and for several years took Blair base posterior and protracto views on all patients. I found that seeing the condyle/atlas accurately is a major challenge with this approach. However, some of the Blair concepts were used to develop the upper cervical analysis and adjustments that I currently use and describe in this book. Taking the Blair seminars gave me greater appreciation for another upper cervical researcher and really expanded my understanding of the upper cervical misalignment.

Then, one day I saw an advertisement for the "Torque Release Technique®" seminar and everything changed again.

"In reality, none of us adjust to restore normal function, but instead, to remove osseous pressure off nerves for restoration of mental impulse supply between brain and body. In turn, then, it is the normal transmission of mental impulse supply which restores normal function. Frequently we are all guilty of emphasizing that which WE DO and of overlooking, or placing in the background, that which INNATE DOES, in the restoration and maintenance of health."

William C. Blair

Torque Release Technique® - TRT

Drs. Marvin Talsky and Jay Holder were both teaching the first Torque Release seminar I attended. I had an associate working for me and we went to the seminar together. When we entered the room, we saw two adjusting tables set up and Dr. Talsky was adjusting people. My associate got on a table. To my surprise, Dr. Talsky soon was adjusting the same subluxations I had found using x-ray and instrumentation.

There was also a salesman at the back of the seminar, promoting surface EMG equipment. The second day, I arrived early and asked the salesman to show me the equipment. He also ran a scan on me.

During a break, I had Dr. Talsky examine me. I have always been a chiropractic challenge and nearly laughed when the examination took longer than usual. Finally, I was adjusted and although I had no complaint I did think I felt better.   Next, I announced that I had been scanned in the morning and I wanted a post adjustment scan. My initial scan showed a large difference in muscle activity at L5-sacrum with the right side above normal and the left side nearly normal. After the adjustment, both sides were nearly equal but both were well beyond the normal range.

I don't think anyone knew what to make of it until I told them that I have a grade 2 spondylo of L5 on sacrum. Innate was pulling both sides equally to hold L5 and sacrum together.

TRT uses The Integrator™, an adjusting instrument, which is a handheld instrument capable of delivering both clockwise and counter-clockwise torque. I began using TRT and the pressure tests I describe were largely a result of this seminar. I found that my results were better when I used x-ray to determine the misalignment rather than trusting the pressure tests alone.

I have heard it said, "If in doubt – adjust." Those are the words of a manipulator.

The TRT notes say, "When in doubt, don't." that is a statement we should all adopt.

At TRT, Network Spinal Analysis was recommended. So I soon found myself at one of Dr. Donald Epstein's seminars.

"Factual evidence upon which proof is established can be reached ONLY by eliminating all variables and establishing constants."

B. J. Palmer

Network Spinal Analysis

Dr. Donald Epstein is developer of Network Spinal Analysis. He provides an information packed seminar and has classified subluxations as class A and class B. Class A subluxations are the classic structural subluxations. Class B subluxations are associated with adverse mechanical cord tension – AMCT.

The NSA protocol seeks to reduce chronic facilitation before attempting to adjust class A subluxations. Low force procedures are typically used to correct both classes of subluxation. Indicators for subluxation are evaluated on each visit. If an adjustment is made, the indicators are once again assessed to determine that a reduction was made.

Care is provided in levels, with definite outcomes and patient involvement established for each level. The goals are to allow the practice member to develop new ways of experiencing the spine, and move to new levels of growth and wellness.

The Network Spinal Analysis seminar stretched my concepts of chiropractic care. I saw patients move through somatopsychic waves that appeared to be beyond conscious control.

I attended a hands–on workshop about one month following Dr. Epstein's seminar. It was there that I began to find what I prefer to call areas of electromagnetic dissonance.

As with Torque Release, not enough emphasis is placed on the upper cervical area and specific correction. However, Dr. Epstein is a skilled clinician and I was sufficiently impressed with the low force adjustments to make them a major part of my practice.

"Down thru our years, our purpose has been to see
HOW LITTLE we need do to get MOST results."
B. J. Palmer

Conclusions

You have now been presented with a rational, scientific approach to chiropractic. When you examine patients on every visit to determine whether or not they are subluxated, you improve the odds by only attempting an adjustment when they really need it. If you use the leg check system as part of your post adjustment examination, you will know that sometimes what you thought were adjustments in fact were not. If you add temperature scans to the leg check, you will find that sometimes leg checks are clear but the temperatures are not. You will then improve the odds some more. Finally, when you are confident that the leg check and the temperature scans are clear you will know that the patient is not subluxated and it is time to let Innate do Its part – and keep your hands off!

Whether you practice upper cervical or Logan basic the approach is still valid. Examine to determine if adjustment is necessary. Adjust if necessary. Then do a post adjustment examination to determine that the adjustment has indeed been made. The approach alone will improve the odds no matter what technique you use.

Finally, even though I began this book by saying that this is a simplified method of analysis, some will argue that other tests are better than the leg checks and temperature scans. Some will argue that there are better ways of taking and analyzing films. Some will argue that there are better ways of delivering adjustments. My reply is – prove it! At least we will be arguing about chiropractic. When the argument is over, the research has been done and we know what really is right – the patient will be the winner! Which was the reason for improving the odds in the first place.

Resources For Continuing - *Improving The Odds*

Seminars
Atlas Orthogonal Technique
        www.atlasorthogonality.com
        The Sweat Clinic
        3274 Buckeye Rd., NE
        Atlanta, GA 30341
        770-457-4430

Blair
        www.blairchiropracticsoc.org
        Convergence
        43931 Division St.
        Lancaster, CA 93535
        404-943-0217 Dr. Brown

Gonstead
        Gonstead Seminars
        www.gonsteadseminar.com
        PO box 3046
        Barrington, IL 60011
        800-842-6852

Grostic/Orthospinology
        www.orthospinology.org
        Dr. Kirk Eriksen
        2500 Flowers Chapel Rd.
        Dothan, AL 36305
        334-793-7992

National Upper Cervical Chiropractic Association (NUCCA)
        www.nucca.org
        Dennis P. Allen, CPA
        Executive Director
        Professional Arts Building
        121 W. Locust St., Suite 208
        Davenport, IA 52803 319-322-7486

Network Spinal Analysis
        www.Donaldepstein.com or www.innateintelligence.com
        444 N. Main St.
        Longmont, CO 80501 303-678-8086

PST

    Chirp Chiropractic Sales, Inc.
    195 S Westmont #L
    Altamonte Springs, FL 32714 800-682-1011

    www.stillwagon.com
    Stillwagon Seminars, Inc.
    767 Dry Run Road
    Monongahela, PA 15063 724-258-6553

Torque Release Technique
    www.torquerelease.com
    Holder Research Institute, Inc.
    3303 Flamingo Drive
    Miami Beach, FL 33140

Books

Herbst, Roger, W., *Gonstead Chiropractic Science & Art* (Sci-Chi Publications, 1980)

Palmer, B. J., *The Subluxation Specific - The Adjustment Specific* (Davenport, IA: The Palmer School of Chiropractic, 1934)

Palmer, D. D., *The Science, Art and Philosophy of Chiropractic* (Portland, OR: Portland Printing House Company, 1910)

Pierce, Walter Vernon, *Results* (Dravosburg, PA: X-Cellent X-Ray Company, 1986)

Stephenson, R. W., *Chiropractic Text Book* (Davenport, IA: The Palmer School of Chiropractic, 1948)

About The Author

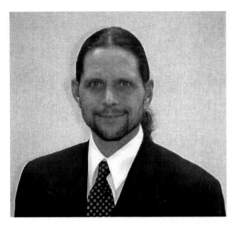

Robert Clyde Affolter

4164 Meridian, Suite 310
Bellingham, WA 98226-5583
360-671-1020 e-mail affolterrc@aol.com

Personal

Age: 47 Birth date: 01/19/55 Height: 5'10" Weight: 160 Race: White
Family: married 23 years
      spouse - Madeline (Mandy) Rene Affolter
      children - Sam (22), Ben (18), Matt (16), Melissa (13)

Education
Diplomas Granted
Doctor of Chiropractic (cum laude), Palmer College of Chiropractic, 1984
Master of Business Administration, University of Kansas, 1978
Bachelor of Arts (chemistry), University of Kansas, 1977
Independence High School, 1973
Certificates Awarded (Professional)
License granted State of Washington, 1985
License granted State of Iowa, 1984
Proficiency, Chiropractic X-ray, Palmer College of Chiropractic, 1984
Passed, The National Board of Chiropractic Examiners, 1984
Proficiency, Grostic, Palmer College of Chiropractic, 1984
Proficiency, PST Advanced, Palmer College of Chiropractic, 1983
Proficiency, Logan Basic, Palmer College of Chiropractic, 1983

Work Experience
President
ChiropractiComplements, Inc., Bellingham, WA
2001 - present

Chiropractor and president
Chiropractic First!, A Professional Service Corporation, Bellingham, WA
1985 - present (sole proprietorship from 1985-1992)

Lecturer
Highline Community College, Des Moines, WA
Spring, 1997

Lecturer
College of Business and Economics, Western Washington University
Bellingham, WA
October, 1984 - June, 1985

Lecturer
Palmer College of Chiropractic, Davenport, IA
July, 1983 - September, 1984

Associate systems engineer
IBM, Topeka, KS
August, 1978 to September, 1981

Author

Author, Improving The Odds, From The Crapshoot Of Manipulative Therapy To The Innate Chiropractic Adjustment, Self-published, 2002
Co-author, Moments of Wisdom, A Guide to Self-Counseling, Writers Club Press, 2000
Articles for *The Chiropractic Journal*, 2001
Articles for *The New Times*, 2000-2001
Articles for *Bellingham Business Journal*, 1996

Inventions

Neck preserver
Oscillemitter
Adjust and rest chiropractic table

CPSIA information can be obtained at www.ICGtesting.com
Printed in the USA
BVOW052216020412

286658BV00004B/1/P

9 780974 586670